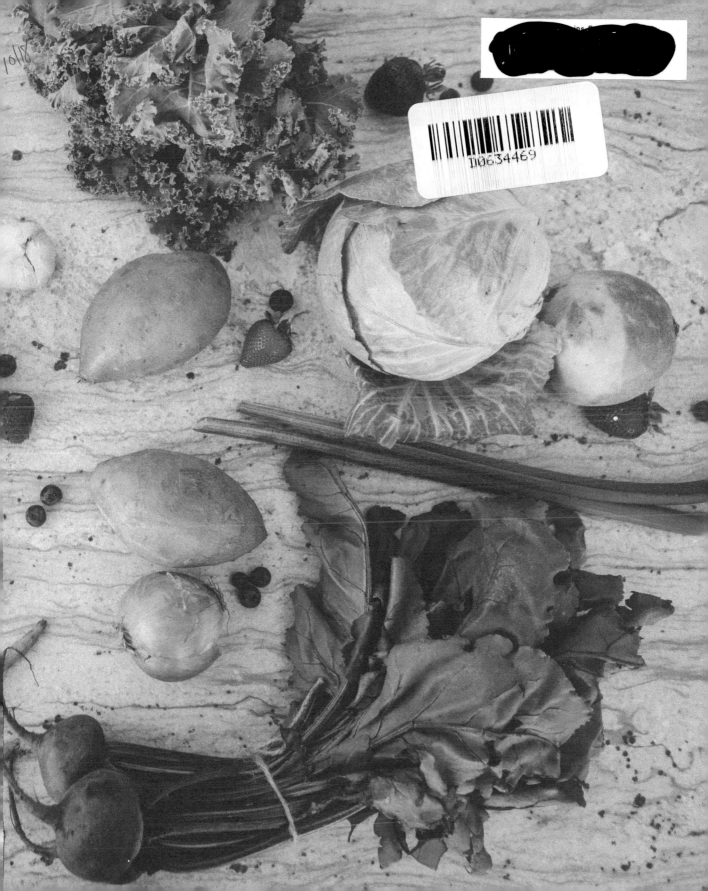

BREAKWATER
P.O. Box 2188, St. John's, NL, Canada, A1C 6E6
WWW.BREAKWATERBOOKS.COM

A CIP catalogue record for this book is available from Library and Archives Canada.
Copyright © 2018 Jessica Mitton
ISBN 978-1-55081-743-0

Canadä

Newfoundland Labrador

We acknowledge the financial support of the Government of Canada and the Government of Newfoundland and Labrador through the Department of Tourism, Culture, Industry and Innovation for our publishing activities.
PRINTED AND BOUND IN CANADA.

Breakwater Books is committed to choosing papers and materials for our books that help to protect our environment. To this end, this book is printed on a recycled paper that is certified by the Forest Stewardship Council®.

SOME GOOD

NUTRITIOUS NEWFOUNDLAND DISHES

Jessica Mitton

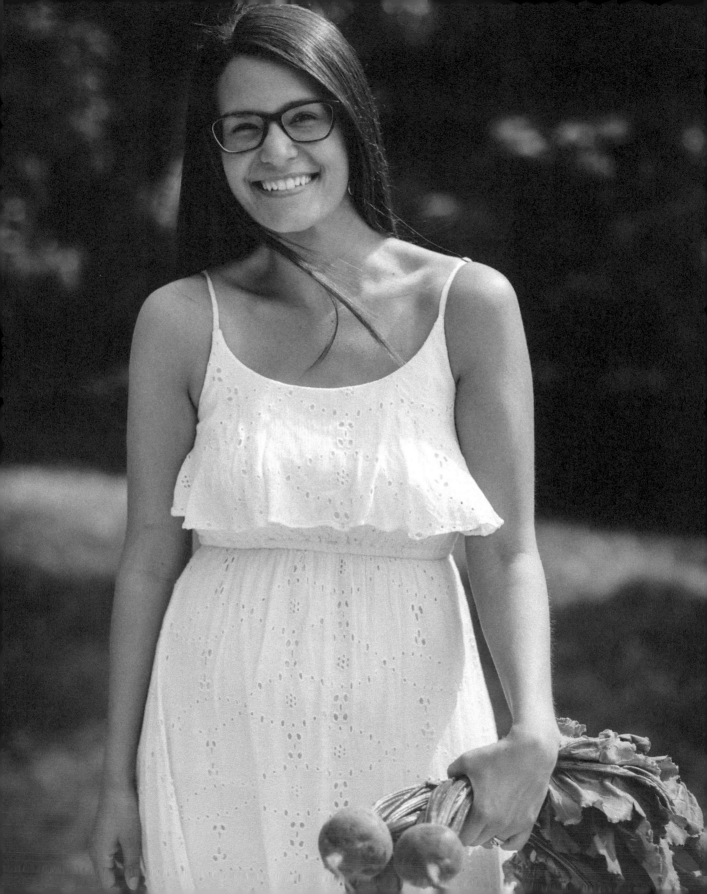

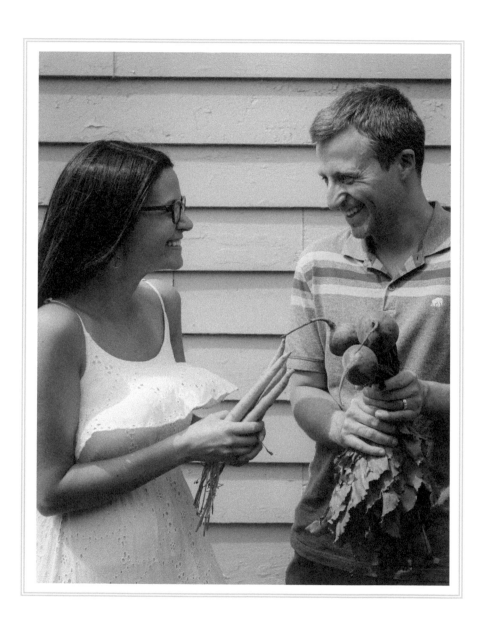

THIS BOOK IS for all the beautiful souls who want to learn about how food really is our medicine, nourishing our bodies throughout our lives. I would like to dedicate it to the memory of our beloved Rudolph, and give thanks to all the people who have made this book possible.

First, to my husband, Gareth, for his ongoing love and support, for being my recipe guinea pig, and for his writing and editing skills (and helping me improve my own). Thanks to my parents, Paul and Daphne. Their support and feedback really helped me develop recipes that actually taste good. Thanks to my big sister, Angela. She drove me to deeply scrutinize my nutritional findings. Thanks to my grandmother, Myrtle, for sharing stories of how Newfoundlanders used to prepare food in the challenging years gone by. Thanks to my grandfather, Paul. His passion for hunting and fishing has always helped ensure that a 'feed' of wild Newfoundland foods was never far from the table. Thanks to Becki Peckham for taking such beautiful photos. Thanks to Jon Payne and Jordan Fowler for letting me invade their space for the photo shoot. Thanks to Heather Stuckless-Haggett for your guidance on the cover design.

Thanks to the amazing team at Breakwater Books for your belief, support, and guidance in bringing this cookbook to life.

Thanks to you all. I hope you enjoy the recipes and the read.

In love and health,

jessica

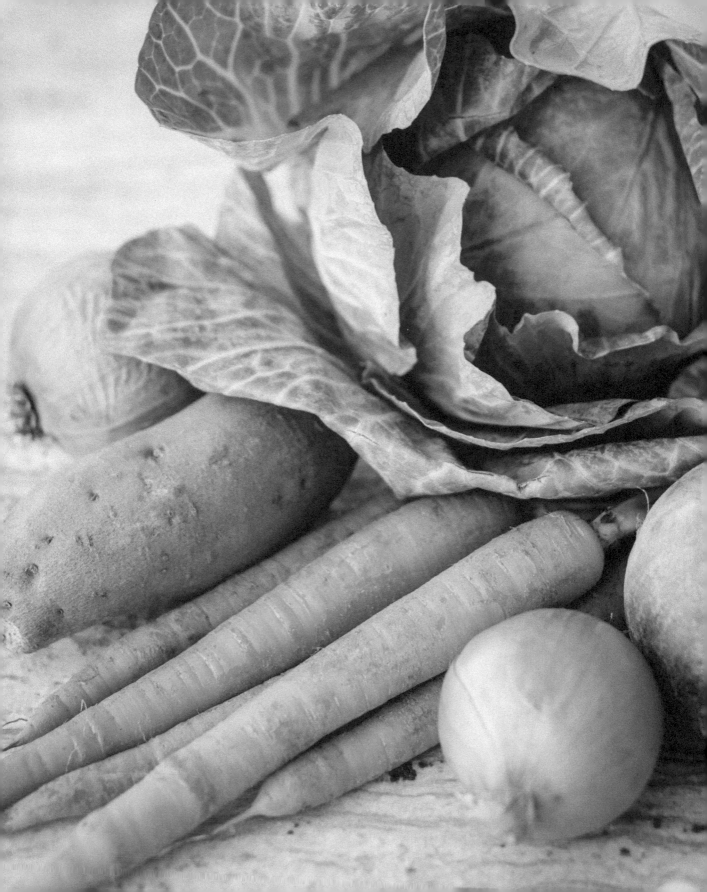

CODFISH AND SALT MEAT: RAISED ON A NEWFOUNDLAND DIET

AS A NATIVE OF THE RURAL WONDERLAND THAT IS GROS MORNE National Park, on Newfoundland's west coast, I was blessed to grow up surrounded by many fresh, local ingredients. My parents cooked with wild moose and salmon, fresh local seafood, and lots of fresh vegetables and fruits. I was actively engaged in foraging for food, venturing out with my parents to pick fresh local berries. Berry picking was great fun. Even though more of my berries made it directly into my mouth than into my bucket, there was always plenty in Mom's and Dad's buckets when we got home!

While the ingredients were often fresh and local, the traditional means of preparation weren't always as healthy as they could have been. Fresh Atlantic cod would often be coated in a wheat-flour-based batter and fried or served up as cod au gratin, soaked in cow's milk and lathered in cheese. Dad's delectable smelling fresh-baked bread was made from refined wheat flour. Homemade baked beans were made using fancy molasses and store-bought condiments that contained many preservatives and additives. Even those fresh berries I helped forage were often used in baked goods filled with refined sugars and wheat flours, or sugary preserves. Perhaps my eating habits growing up weren't as beneficial for my body as they could have been, considering I was raised in a place so abundant in fresh local ingredients.

What's not in doubt is that my eating habits didn't improve when I became an adult, flew the nest, and life got busier. Suddenly, I had no one to lovingly prepare meals for me, and gradually, I tended towards the convenience foods that were quick, easy, and abundant in the city. Today, I see more and more of these quick-and-easy convenience foods becoming available while, at the same time, our cooking habits are not always what they could be.

As I started to learn about nutrition and the ways food affects our bodies, I began to get creative in the kitchen. After obtaining my Holistic Nutritional Consultant certification, I decided I wanted to learn how to cook and bake foods I love while making them nourishingly delicious. At that point, I enrolled in another course to become a Culinary Nutrition Expert. This provided me with the skills I needed to turn some old favourites into nourishingly delicious new dishes that would be acceptable for the improved standards I had set for myself. So began what has become an ongoing passion. I am always tweaking recipes and creating new ways to get nourishing foods into my body that taste great, and I'm committed to sharing the fruits of my labour with others so we can all be the healthiest we can be!

I was inspired to write this book because of that deep desire to urge anyone and everyone to get back in the kitchen and cook from scratch. I also wanted to spread the word that the famous traditional Newfoundland dishes we know and love can be reimagined to become more healthy and nourishing, but still *some good*! These are foods, snacks, and meals all Newfoundlanders will know well, whether as everyday fare or occasional go-to comfort foods, and in this book you will discover innovative twists on some of my favourite homemade dishes, along with newly created recipes infused with and inspired by the ingredients I grew up eating.

My goal as a Holistic Nutritional Consultant is to help people live a healthy lifestyle each and every day, and not to focus on conventional or fad diets. By eating local, fresh, and in-season foods, we help to nourish our bodies as optimally as possible, as well as supporting our community and the environment. This book is designed to point you towards the most nutritiously delicious ingredients while still allowing you to enjoy your favourite Newfoundland dishes. It is my hope that these recipes will enable you to incorporate healthier choices the next time you set out to prepare a Newfoundland favourite, as well as starting you off, or guiding you along, on your personal journey to a healthier lifestyle.

I have focused on gluten-free, dairy-free, and refined-sugar-free recipes, as these are the main culprit ingredients that can have negative effects on our health. Working the kinds of recipes outlined in this book into your kitchen, and into your life, will help your body become a little bit cleaner, leaner, and healthier in the long run. Enjoy!

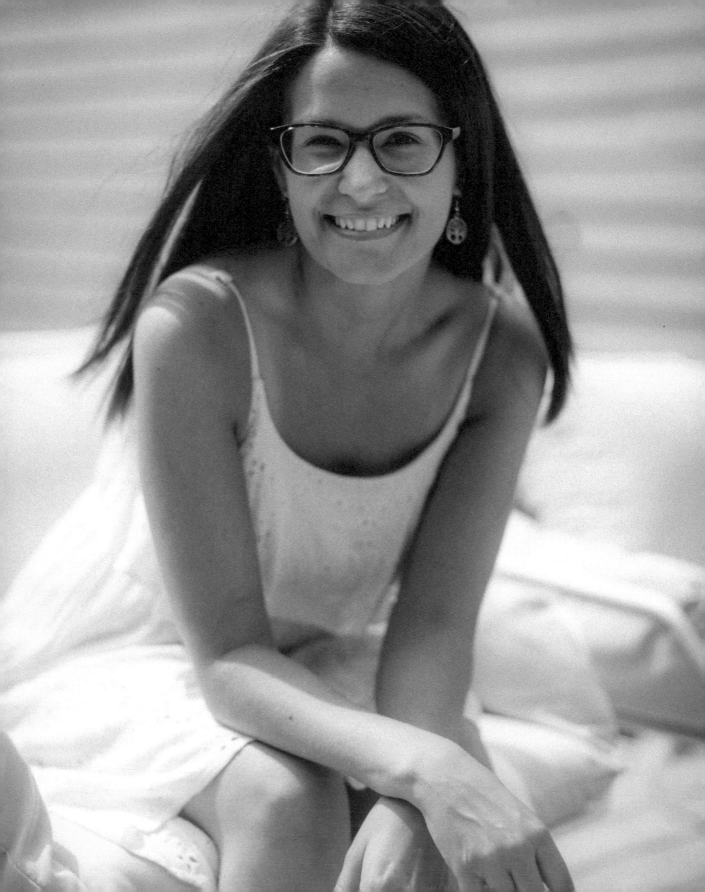

MY JOURNEY TO NUTRITION

TODAY, HOLISTIC AND CULINARY NUTRITION IS MY GREATEST PASSION, but this wasn't always the case. In fact, you might say I've taken the scenic route to discovering my life's purpose. While I did dabble with cooking as a youngster, and even applied to a culinary college when first leaving high school, my life took a very different route. I chose to enrol in university instead, earning a business degree at Memorial University of Newfoundland. (Total opposite to cooking, I know!) I suppose at that time I thought of cooking as a hobby with an unpredictable career path, so I made what I thought was a sensible decision, switched directions, and got my BBA. What I didn't know then is that life isn't about following the money; it's about following your dreams and passions.

By the age of thirty, I'd already had a pretty successful career working with a financial institution. I moved to New Brunswick after finishing my business degree and landed my first 'proper' job. I did quite well there, rising through the ranks and working in several positions; but my fascination with food continued, and I soon discovered a nutrition workshop being offered in my area. At the time, I was suffering with digestive issues and beginning to realize the benefits of eliminating gluten from my diet. I wanted to learn more and was excited to discover a whole program on nutrition that would allow me to become a Certified Holistic Nutritional Consultant™. I enjoyed the workshop so much I decided to enrol in the program, while still working full-time. (Yes, life was busy!)

Towards the end of my time at the financial institution, I was tired, anemic, and overweight. My digestive issues continued. I was stressed and anxious, and was eventually diagnosed with a massive uterine fibroid tumour. I also had a cyst on one of my ovaries and one in my breast.

I decided to move back to Newfoundland to get some family support and started applying for jobs close to home. I was offered a position at another financial institution, so I took it and decided to complete the remainder of my nutrition program online. Unfortunately, my health continued to worsen until something had to be done about my ever-growing fibroid. Despite my best efforts to seek help and advice to treat my condition, the fibroid was out of control, and it became too dangerous for me to wait any longer. I was left with no choice but to undergo surgery. I couldn't believe it! How could somebody still so young require major surgery? I was frustrated and afraid.

So I made a life-changing decision. I quit my job and abandoned a potentially lucrative career in banking to become a Holistic Nutritional Consultant. I wanted to learn more, and I wanted to avoid anything like this ever happening to me again.

I made a vow to myself: No more surgeries, thank you very much! This resonated all the more because my family history was littered with such procedures. The writing was on the wall, and it certainly had my attention. It was a huge wake-up call and set me on a mission to find out what I could do to help myself live a healthy, vibrant, and (hopefully) surgery-free life.

On a personal level, these choices and this wholly new lifestyle have had dramatically positive effects. Now, I truly feel that I am thriving in life, and as a Holistic Nutritional Consultant and Culinary Nutrition Expert, I get to follow my heart and spend my time helping others.

NEWFOUNDLAND ROOTS: A BRIEF HISTORY OF FOOD ON THE ROCK

AS PEOPLE, WE ALL HAVE AN INEXTRICABLE CONNECTION TO FOOD. It nourishes, fuels, and sustains us. Without it, we can't live. It also brings us great pleasure and satiation, as well as being at the centre of many social events and gatherings. Go anywhere in the world and there is a culture around food. Be it the patisseries of Paris, the coffee shops of Rome, or the markets of India, food is front and centre in every corner of the globe.

This connection between people and food is equally apparent in Newfoundland. We are an island province with a rich history of fishing.[1] Still today, our fishers set out on the mighty Atlantic's waves to bring its bounty to shore. In many respects, these people's lives are ordered around the gathering, preparation, and consumption of food. While our larger centres are fully equipped with the big chain take-outs, restaurants, and superstores, the majority of the inhabited island still revolves around decades-old (even centuries-old) fishing communities, many with fishers still hard at work.

But the bounty isn't restricted to the ocean. On land, we have a deep tradition of hunting and snaring. From hulking moose to scurrying

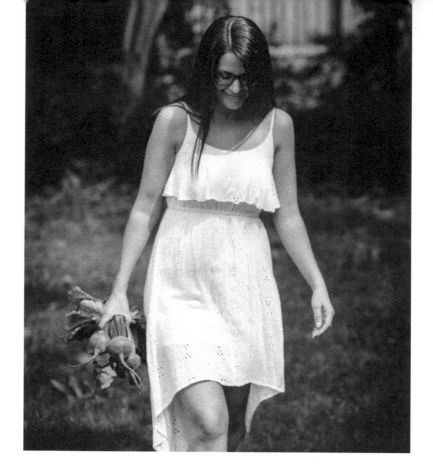

rabbits, our pristine forests are home to a diverse and plentiful selection of wild game, along with colourful berries that burst with distinct flavour and pack a nutritional punch well above their weight. Partridgeberries, bakeapples (also known as cloudberries), blueberries, strawberries, raspberries, and many more grow wildly and prevalently across the island.

Yet despite this cornucopia of available whole and wholesome ingredients, Newfoundlanders' relationship to their food has not always been a happy one. Back in the 1800s, doctors researching health concerns in Newfoundland noted a pervasiveness of tuberculosis, along with diseases directly related to nutrient deficiency, such as scurvy, rickets, and beriberi. They also began to find that malnutrition was one of the greatest medical problems facing Newfoundland and Labrador at the time.[2]

Chief among the causes of these multifarious epidemics were two key factors: insufficient access to food in general and insufficient access to food that was nutrient dense.

As remains the case today, the Newfoundland climate made it very challenging to grow food, with such a limited growing season. This meant that much of the food had to be imported, greatly increasing the cost. Spoilage was another issue, as electricity for fridges and freezers would not become widely available in Newfoundland until the 1950s.

As a result of scarcity and necessity, food choices largely came down to the availability, accessibility, and durability of the food. The limited locally grown options had to be supplemented by foods that could be preserved and foods that had a long shelf life.

This gave rise to a tradition that lives strong in Newfoundland today: preservation. Salting, smoking, pickling, and the use of root cellars became necessary solutions to the food-shortage challenge, and such preserves remain a staple of the traditional Newfoundland diet to this day.

Foods rich in nutrients were slim pickings. There were meat and berries aplenty in the woods, and on the barrens and marshes, but they required foraging or picking, and for hardworking Newfoundlanders, time was at as much of a premium as nutrient-rich foods. Meanwhile, it was difficult to bring in fresh foods from elsewhere, as importation time was long and the food would spoil by the time it reached Newfoundland's shores. Eating foods with a long shelf life helped people feed their families; however, these types of foods lacked the nutrients for their bodies to stay healthy, and in turn, they became malnourished.

The three main health conditions affecting Newfoundlanders of the time could be attributed to a lack of specific nutrients in their limited diets. These were scurvy (lack of vitamin C), rickets (lack of vitamin D), and beriberi (lack of vitamin B1, also known as thiamine).[3]

Malnourishment depletes the immune system, limiting the body's ability to fight off viruses and bacteria. With tuberculosis—an infectious disease affecting the lungs—so prevalent at the time, many Newfoundlanders were unable to fight off the often deadly disorder, which may have to some extent been attributable to malnourishment.[4]

With so many health conditions impacting the Newfoundland population, a number of women trained in nutrition were sent in from the U.S. to teach people about the importance of the food they were consuming in maintaining good health. However, this did little good, for all the education in the world could not make up for the harsh fact that the beneficial food was simply not available to the people in high enough quantities or with any consistency.[5]

In our time of modern convenience, it is difficult to relate to a time when people were becoming sick due to a lack of healthy food. But today, we face a new kind of food problem—here in Newfoundland and around the developed world.

Over time, foods entered a phase of mass production, and evermore inventive ways of packaging, preserving, and distributing food brought a new abundance of edible options to our big-box-store shelves. Many of these foods became enriched or fortified with vitamins. While this has been sold to us as progress and a solution to food lack, we are now discovering that many of the foods we eat today pose problems of their own. Many of the so-called foods that fill our store shelves contain very high amounts of sugar and rancid fats that are detrimental to our health. We are now marketed not real, whole food, but *food-like* products—colourfully packaged, stacked to the ceiling and along sprawling aisles.

The ingredient list of a packaged food item today reveals that what's contained within is not just food. We are faced with lists of unpronounceable artificial flavourings, additives, salt, and sugar (often cleverly disguised under one of its many nom de plumes, such as corn syrup, cane sugar, glucose, fructose, malt syrup, agave—the list goes on). These nasties are added not to improve the nutritional quality of the food, but to make food taste as we expect it to and to keep you coming back for more. The *big three* taste bud-targeting ingredients—salt, sugar, and fat—are dialled up and down in an attempt to target our *bliss point*[6] Through clever combinations of these health-harming ingredients, food producers get us hooked on unnaturally exaggerated flavours that make returning to real food a challenge for millions. By turning up one or two of these ingredients, food producers are able to make claims such as 'low fat,' when in fact many of these food-like products are high in sodium and/or sugar and not very good for us at all.

The result is a modern food system that is in many ways broken, and perhaps worse for our health than in past times of scarcity. We are now seeing numerous health concerns arising that could be prevented with simple good food and nutrition. Conditions such as high blood pressure, allergies, high cholesterol, and type 2 diabetes abound in the Western world, and instead of changing our eating habits, we continue with harmful dietary behaviour and take medications to mask or manage the symptoms. Many of these medications carry side effects of their own, and the whole vicious circle continues.

This may seem like an extreme perspective, but it is only the truth. Think about how many people you know within your own circle of family and friends who are unwell and taking multiple medications. Many of these people could have prevented their plight with better nutritional choices. Many of them could begin to reverse their symptoms and gradually reduce their intake of medications. In my line of work, I have seen this firsthand.

What's the answer? A return to real, whole foods.

We have come such a long way since those days of scarcity and struggle. Today, we are blessed like never before with technology to bring the right foods into our homes and keep them fresh for longer. We have electricity, refrigerators, freezers, and proper ways to store our foods. We have easy, convenient access to foods that will keep us healthy. We have better methods of preserving our foods that can themselves provide us with health benefits, such as fermentation. We have the tools to prepare healthy and delicious meals. We have access to education that will teach us about the importance of our diet to our overall health, wellbeing, and quality of life. Let's do it right this time, heeding the lessons of the past, putting our greater nutritional knowledge to good use, and taking full advantage of the myriad resources at hand.

In the past, Newfoundlanders suffered from malnutrition through no fault of their own. Today, many of us are malnourished simply due to a lack of understanding about what we are putting inside of ourselves, or a failure to take responsibility for the fuel we provide to our bodies. Neither of these is necessary or justifiable.

Bad rancid fats, sugar, additives, and refined foods—including wheat and dairy products—may feed our hunger and satisfy our taste buds, but they do nothing for our health. In a sense, we are starving ourselves when we eat these food-like products—starving our bodies of nourishment, and overburdening our systems with toxic substances. But we now have the resources and the knowledge to turn things around and get ourselves healthy again.

This book will help you along the path to nutritious food made from real, whole ingredients, with some distinctly Newfoundland dishes created in ways that are nourishingly delicious!

NEWFOUNDLAND'S BOUNTY: NOURISHING FOODS FROM OUR SEAS AND SHORES

THE FISH

WHEN WE THINK OF NEWFOUNDLAND FOODS, FRESH SEAFOOD IS THE first thing that comes to mind. Our connection to the ocean and its bounty is woven into the history and culture of our island home. Coastal communities adorn almost every bay around Newfoundland's rugged coast, most of which were built on fishing, and many of which are still home to fishers today.

Back in the day, the salt-cod fishery was a major Newfoundland industry, often with entire families participating in the process of curing the fresh catch. While the cod fishery may have seen its ups and downs over the years, it remains a part of the heart and soul of this place, and we are lucky to still be able to access this succulent fish today. Not only is fresh Atlantic codfish dense, flaky, and delicious, it is also packed with many great nutrients, including vitamin B12, iodine, and omega-3.[7]

Salmon is another fish that is a Newfoundland staple, fished as far back as the days of the Beothuk—Newfoundland's Indigenous people—and still fished here today.[8] Add to the list trout, scallops, shrimp, lobster, Arctic char, and more, and it is plain to see that we Newfoundlanders are truly blessed to have such a health-giving ocean and freshwater bounty at our disposal.

WILD MOOSE MEAT

Moose may be common in Newfoundland these days, but they are not native to the province. They were introduced in 1904, when just four moose were introduced to provide food and sport.[9] The lack of a primary predator and the ideal habitat of the island's boreal forest have allowed moose to thrive, so hunters are permitted to hunt these large animals in the fall of each year, and moose meat makes its way to many Newfoundland dinner tables, prepared in a variety of ways.

Moose meat is in fact a good meat to eat, for a number of reasons. Because moose are herbivores, chowing down on plants, trees, and shrubs, and since they live in the wild, there are none of the concerns that often arise around farmed animals. We can rest assured that our wild-caught moose meat has not been injected with any growth hormones or antibiotics. Moose is also a lean meat that does not have a high fat content. Rich in vitamins, including some of the B vitamins—niacin (B3) and B2—as well as some great minerals, including selenium, iron, and zinc, eating a 'feed' of moose will surely give you some health benefits.[10]

Some of the favoured ways of eating moose include moose stew, moose sausages, oven roasted, or my Dad's preferred way—sliced and fried in a pan with onions and a little salt and pepper. I can smell it now!

VEGETABLES

Potatoes, potatoes, potatoes! Newfoundland has always had an abundance of them. As a result, this hardy root has starred in Newfoundland culture for many years—a food staple that has been

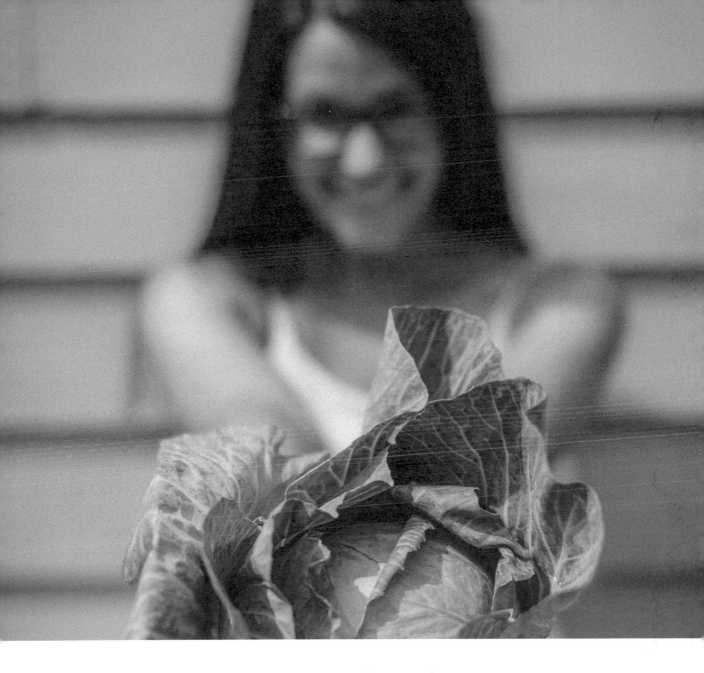

incorporated into dishes across the province and across its history. Potatoes and other vegetables were grown to supplement the fishery, and it is probably difficult for many traditionalists to contemplate their meals minus those hearty white potatoes. In this cookbook, however, you will notice I replace white potato with sweet potato. Not only do

I personally enjoy the flavour of a sweet potato over that of a white potato, but its nutrient profile is also a little higher than that of the white potato. (If you are looking for a dose of vitamin A, you won't go without when you eat a sweet potato!) Also, anytime you eat the bright colours of the rainbow, that's how you know you are getting a higher dose of some very important phytochemicals as well.[11]

Let's not forget, though, that there are lots of other root vegetables to choose from. Turnip and carrot are still firmly on the menu, as well as everyone's favourite leafy cruciferous vegetable, the cabbage. Or, in other words, the remaining vegetables that make up that most famous of Newfoundland dishes, Jiggs Dinner. I hope you like my twist on this legendary dish, my Jiggs Dinner Veggie Cakes recipe. I created this recipe without boiling any vegetables, as boiling for long periods of time can remove many of the nutrients and leave them behind in the water, meaning they never make it to do their good work in our bodies. Baking, roasting, or steaming these lovely, nutrient-dense vegetables are great ways to optimize your nutritional hit when enjoying them for or with your next meal.

Onion is another great vegetable often found on Newfoundland dinner plates. It has been used in the dressings that stuff our turkeys, to make those *de-lish* fish cakes, and to fry up with a bit of moose meat. Onion is one of the key ingredients that infuses our Newfoundland dishes with their trademark flavour, and I've made plentiful use of onions in the recipes.

BOUNTIFUL BERRIES

Berries grow in all corners of Newfoundland, and these colourful gems offer us a deep and diverse nutrient profile. Their flavours range from bitter to sour and sweet. You could call berries Newfoundland's natural candy. Blueberries, partridgeberries, bakeapples, raspberries, dewberries, and the many more edible berries of our province add flavour to our favourite baked goods, preserves, and snacks. With some amazing antioxidant and nutritional properties, eating berries can be as beneficial as it is enjoyable. Antioxidants help prevent damage from the free-radical activity happening all the time in our bodies. Free radicals are molecules that become oxidized and can cause damage to our tissues if they are not balanced with antioxidants.[12] Some other great nutrients found in berries include vitamin C, fibre, potassium, and magnesium, among many others.[13]

SAVOURY

Savoury is an herb found in many traditional Newfoundland dishes, including our fish cakes, dressing, and seasoning for a roast chicken or turkey. As well as tasting great, savoury offers many wonderful nutrients, including magnesium, iron, and vitamin A.[14]

Can you see a pattern emerging here? This province offers plenty of foods with the nutrients to optimally fuel our bodies, and taste amazing while doing it. When we take a closer look at processed foods like white sugar, refined wheat flours, and processed dairy products, we see that so many of the nutrients are stripped away, and all the processing these foods go through leaves them devoid of many of their natural vitamins and minerals. Many times, the vitamins and minerals you see listed on the nutrition label are synthetically added after the initial processing. (Milk is a perfect example of this.)

Every body needs the natural nutrients from real, whole food in order to work in an optimal state and stay healthy. For example, calcium is great for our bones, magnesium is important for our muscles, and vitamin C supports the immune system. It's important to get these nutrients in their natural state to ensure you are getting good-quality nutrition and a variety of nutrients so they can work together, support each other, and keep you ticking along. Processing and refining our foods only serves to deplete their nutrients, therefore depleting our bodies. Focusing on the whole foods available to us will help us feed our bodies with the natural nutrients found in nature.

LIVING WITHOUT DAIRY, GLUTEN, AND REFINED SUGAR

FOR MANY PEOPLE, IN NEWFOUNDLAND AND OTHER PARTS OF THE Western world, an examination of their average, day-to-day diet would reveal pretty high amounts of these ingredients. Gluten is in many foods, including pastas, breads, crackers, seasonings, and spice mixes. Dairy is everywhere, from the colourful cartons of multifariously processed milks in most everybody's fridge, to yogurt, coffee creamers, and in many places we might not think of, such as pureed soups. Refined sugar appears in the obvious places, like candy bars, and the less obvious, like ketchup and—believe it or not—that milk you are pouring on your breakfast cereal or chugging by the glass-load.

Part of discovering my new healthy lifestyle through food involved cutting out dairy, gluten, and refined sugar. By eliminating these three ingredients that are so pervasive in the average modern-day diet, and instead focusing on eating wholefoods, I've seen amazing results and improvements to my overall health.

DAIRY

Dairy really is everywhere. It gives soups their creaminess; soaks breakfast cereals; adorns pizzas, pasta dishes, tacos, and many more common meals; shows up as a tempting yogurt parfait; or appears as the seemingly harmless creamer in your coffee. When you consider its myriad guises, most people might consider living without dairy to be almost unfathomable. Well, you can capture that creamy taste and texture without needing to consume dairy. But why would you want to remove dairy in the first place, you might ask?

There are a number of reasons why we might all want to get over milk. Chief among them is Bovine Growth Hormone (rBGH). While this hormone does not affect milk production in Canada (it has thankfully been banned here), it is legal to use in the United States. (There are, however, hormonal growth promoters that are given to beef cattle in Canada.[15]) rBGH increases a hormone in cows in order to supercharge their milk production. While the cows may produce more milk, this unnatural fiddling with their hormones also makes them more prone to infections, hence requiring the use of antibiotics.[16] All of this will find its way into the milk they are producing, so that 'fresh' milk in those colourful cartons may not be exactly as it's been marketed to us.

The harsh reality is that, despite their engineered 'healthful' reputation, dairy products such as milk, cheese, and yogurt are just more examples of the highly refined and processed food items that abound in our grocery stores. After milk has been retrieved from a cow, it is then stored, transported, lab tested, pasteurized, homogenized, and separated—and that's just the milk itself.[17] Further processing will then occur if the milk is to be used for yogurt or cheese products. In addition, many substances are added to milk and dairy products to make them taste better, including refined sugar and synthetic vitamins.

As with gluten, dairy products can cause many issues in people who are unable to break down some of its components, such as the sugar and proteins of milk. The sugar in milk is known as lactose, while the proteins are called casein and whey. In order to break down lactose so our bodies can use it properly, we need an enzyme called lactase. Unfortunately, as we progress into adulthood and get older, some people become less able to produce this enzyme. This is why we see so many people who are lactose intolerant, and this inability to break down lactose can cause various issues, such as bloating, abdominal discomfort, and diarrhoea.[18]

But we all know that dairy is an excellent source of calcium, right? Well, not so much. While dairy products may contain some calcium, they aren't necessarily the best source of calcium, as we have been led to believe. Dairy products are alkalizing before being processed; however, once they are processed and metabolized in our bodies, they become acidifying. Therefore, when we consume a dairy product, it has an acidifying affect, and our bodies need to pull from our vitamin and mineral stores in order to deal with it. Maintaining an acid-alkaline balance in our body is very important. If we become too acidic, our bodies become more prone to health issues.[19] In addition, because dairy products are highly processed, the actual amount of calcium left is questionable. The processing strips a lot of the natural calcium, and calcium is often later synthetically added. Wholefood sources of calcium are a much safer bet, with the added advantage of having a less acidifying effect on our bodies. Some rich wholefood sources of calcium to reach for way before milk include kale, spinach, collard greens, sesame seeds, and almonds.

This news may be hard for some to swallow, so ingrained in our collective consciousness is the link between milk and strong bones, but it's time to dispel the milk-calcium myth we've all been fed by the powerful dairy industry and advertisers. It sure has shifted a lot of colourful cartons, but dairy quite simply is far from the best source of calcium out there.

DAIRY ALTERNATIVES

NUT AND SEED MILKS

Nut and seed milks are an awesome alternative to dairy. When making them from scratch, you get the added benefit of avoiding the additives that can find their way into store-bought nut and seed milks. Nuts and seeds have so many nutrients, and by soaking them overnight you just make those nutrients so much more available.

Here is my Almond Milk recipe for you to try. It's great to use as a dairy-milk alternative.

ALMOND MILK

YIELDS 2 LITRES

PREP TIME: overnight + 10 minutes

2 cups almonds, soaked overnight
8 cups water
2 tsp honey
2 tsp vanilla extract

1 Rinse soaked almonds.

2 Blend soaked almonds, water, honey, and vanilla extract until smooth. You may have to do this in batches according to the size of your blender.

3 Pour almond liquid through milk bag and strain out the pulp. Store in a Mason jar for up to four days.

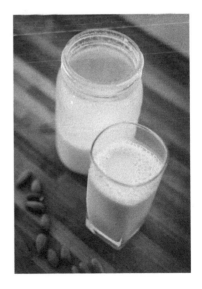

GLUTEN

Gluten has been getting a lot of attention in recent years, and not in a good way. In fact, *gluten free* has become a trending food topic that has penetrated mainstream consciousness and, as a result, our grocery-store shelves, restaurants, and eateries. When these trends come along, a couple of things happen. First, many people begin trying to eradicate the said food product from their diets just because it's trendy, without really understanding the benefits of doing so. Later, widespread cynicism sets in, the trend becomes labelled a fad, and many people laugh it off as an irrelevance. So, what's the truth about gluten? Is it something we should fear and try to avoid, or is it just the latest trendy topic of our food-fad culture?

The fact of the matter is that eating gluten-free can have many positive effects on the average person's health. While some are more obviously allergic to gluten than others, many people would benefit from eradicating gluten from their diet. But let's back up for a second and talk about what exactly gluten is.

Gluten is a protein found in wheat, rye, and barley.[20] It acts as the 'glue' in dishes or foods that include these ingredients, giving them their form and substance. Gluten is most commonly found in foods like pastries, breads, bagels, and cereals. However, it can often be found hiding in other, less obvious places, such as salad dressings, sauces, alcoholic beverages, and even beauty products.

While gluten may appear in many foods that most people consume on a daily basis, that doesn't mean it is good for you. People may think that eating gluten-free constitutes a diet, similar to counting calories or eating paleo; however, it is the view of the holistic nutrition community that there is no such thing as *a diet*—only *your diet.* The concept of 'dieting' is the result of marketing campaigns that encourage short-term (often intrinsically unhealthy) ways of eating, or consuming chemical-laden food substitutes. This concept is rooted in a quick-fix mentality, and even those who successfully lose weight following the rules of a trendy diet often do so in an unhealthy way, and often return to unhealthy eating and lifestyle habits once they reach a specific goal—usually a weight goal. This is neither a healthy, nor a sustainable approach, and it is much better to commit to understanding the way your food—your fuel—interacts with your body, and to maintaining a healthy, balanced approach to eating (and living!) over the long term.

Eating gluten-free is not a diet, and neither is eliminating just gluten from your diet a wondrous fix-all for your health issues. Rather, the act of eliminating gluten from your diet is an advisable part of pursuing an overall healthy lifestyle. Gluten-free is not a fad; consuming it can be a genuine cause for concern.

There are many reasons why consuming gluten can be harmful for your health. For those suffering with celiac disease, the effects are more immediate. Celiac is an autoimmune disease that necessitates complete avoidance of gluten consumption, as it causes damage to the small intestine in the sufferer.[21] But those with celiac disease aren't the only ones who should be giving gluten a miss. Many people have a degree of sensitivity to gluten. As Holistic Nutritional Consultants, we understand that no two people are the same when it comes to the effects of the things we consume. There are those who are not celiac, but nonetheless very gluten-sensitive. For these people, consuming any amount of gluten will cause issues and discomfort. The reason for this is that gluten can make your intestinal wall weak or permeable, allowing minute particles to pass into the bloodstream.[22] This can cause allergies and a host of other problems, and there is plenty of research demonstrating this common sensitivity and its effects.[23] Some symptoms and conditions that may result from gluten sensitivity include bloating, abdominal pain, abnormal bowel habits, joint pain, foggy mind, headaches, anxiety, neurological dysfunction, and skin conditions.

Therefore, it is quite possible you could be suffering from any of the above symptoms due to an undiagnosed gluten allergy. Of course, if you have a nasty rash or an unrelenting headache, you need to get checked out by a medical doctor, but many M.D.s won't check for a gluten allergy, or advise a patient not to eat bread or other gluten-heavy foods. By talking to a nutritionist or naturopath, or experimenting with the foods you eat and avoid, you can decipher if a chronic problem can be traced to gluten; however, reducing the gluten in one's diet can be a good idea for many people.

So, we've established that gluten-free is not a fad and that eradicating gluten from our diets can be beneficial for many, and we've looked at some of the negative effects that result from eating gluten. But since gluten is in a lot of foods, how can we enjoy the foods we like without consuming all that gluten? The good news is there are alternatives. One benefit of the recent popularizing of the gluten subject is that you can find gluten-free information and recipes easily, online and in bookstores. Similarly, this book is filled with recipes that can help introduce a gluten-free approach to your Newfoundland-inspired dishes. In addition, there are many other types of flours you can use as an alternative to wheat, rye, and barley, so you can prepare and enjoy foods like your favourite baked goodies in a new, healthier way. Let's have a look at some of the gluten-free flours I enjoy using, to get you started.

FLOUR ALTERNATIVES

There are so many options when trying to stay away from flours that contain gluten. When baking, I have discovered that the best results often come from mixing a number of gluten-free flours together to get an ideal blend. Not only does this approach offer a flavour mixture that prevents the taste of one flour from overwhelming the flavour of your food, it also maximizes the properties of each of the flours, so your flour blend works optimally for the specific dish you are preparing. When cooking, I tend to stick with one flour, as cooking doesn't require such large amounts as baking. The options are endless! Try out some of these flours to replace your wheat, rye, or barley next time you bake or cook.

BUCKWHEAT FLOUR

Buckwheat flour is created simply by grinding buckwheat. Don't be confused by the name—even though it has the word *wheat* in it, there is no actual wheat in this flour. It has an earthy, nutty flavour, it's a good source of fibre, and it's a great flour to use for baking. Pancakes, anyone?

BROWN RICE FLOUR

Brown rice flour is made simply by grinding brown rice. This flour is a good source of fibre and manganese, and has a mild nutty flavour. It's very versatile and great to use for both cooking and baking.

ALMOND FLOUR

Almond flour is made simply by—you guessed it—grinding almonds. Want another astounding insight? It tastes like almonds! This flour is a great source of magnesium and fibre. I prefer to combine almond flour with other flours when baking; though it can be used on its own

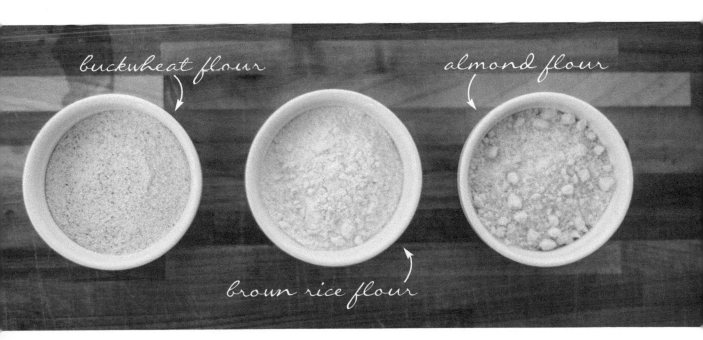

buckwheat flour

almond flour

brown rice flour

provided you don't mind that almond flavour coming through. Almond flour also makes for a perfect breadcrumb substitute, and I like to use it as a delicious, crispy, gluten-free batter when cooking!

COCONUT FLOUR
Coconut flour has a light coconut taste and is another good source of fibre. This is another one I prefer to use in a blend with other flours when baking.

TEFF FLOUR
Teff flour is made from the very tiny teff grain. It's a great source of calcium and fibre and is perfect for use in baking recipes.

MILLET FLOUR
Millet is packed with protein and has a mild flavour. You can use millet when baking or cooking.

QUINOA FLOUR
Quinoa flour is great to use, as quinoa is a complete protein, meaning it contains an adequate proportion of all nine of the essential amino acids necessary for the dietary needs of human beings. While quinoa flour can be used for both baking and cooking, it is best mixed with other flours, as it has a very distinct nutty flavour that can be a little overpowering.

ARROWROOT FLOUR/STARCH
Arrowroot is mostly used as a thickening agent for sauces, soups, or stews; however, it can be used in flour blends too.

SORGHUM FLOUR
Sorghum is a grain that is ground into flour. It's great for both baking and cooking. It has a very mild taste with the added benefit of being high in protein and antioxidants.

TAPIOCA FLOUR

Tapioca flour—also known as tapioca starch—is made from the cassava plant. This flour does not have any distinct taste and is great for thickening sauces, soups, or stews. You can also use it for baking, but it is best used in combination with other flours.

GARBANZO BEAN FLOUR

Garbanzo bean flour is also known as chickpea flour, as that's what it's made from. Unsurprisingly for a flour made from chickpeas, it's a great source of protein and fibre. While garbanzo flour can be used for both baking and cooking, when baking, it is best combined with other flours.

OAT FLOUR

Oat flour is made simply by grinding oats and is a great source of fibre and manganese. It's a good flour to use in baked goods and gluten-free breads when combined with other flours.

REFINED SUGAR

Refined sugar has been shown in numerous studies to have addictive properties.[24] Did you also know that cane sugar has to go through multiple steps to eventually become the granulated white sugar that can be purchased at the store? The refining process is very extensive, leaving the white sugar you buy with only one remaining nutrient—a lonely carbohydrate. Refined sugar is in everything from your baked goods to the ketchup and milk stored in your refrigerator. Today, we are constantly exposed to sugar consumption through a multitude of different foods, often without even realizing we are eating it.

Think brown sugar is a healthier alternative? Think again. Brown sugar is essentially the same as refined white sugar. It has been through just as many steps of processing and has just as little to offer in terms of nutritional value. The only real difference is the colour, which brown sugar gets from molasses. While there may be a few trace minerals from the molasses, brown sugar is nonetheless still a highly refined sugar and sticking solely to unrefined sugar alternatives is the nutrient-conscious way to go.

It isn't only this standard sugar that is highly refined, either. So too are the refined white flours and breads that litter (and that's a good word for it, because this stuff is garbage) our store shelves. Not only do these foods provide us with zero nutrients, but they actively deplete our bodies of important nutrients.[25] Our taste buds have been hijacked and conditioned over time, to the point that we now crave or desire that sweet tasting beverage or baked dessert on a daily basis. So how do we get ourselves out of this vicious cycle? Simply, by getting back to making our food from scratch, using real ingredients. Understanding and controlling the types and amounts of sugars you use in your dishes will help keep your body healthy.

How does the nasty, refined white (or brown) stuff really affect our health? Here's how:

Nutrient Deficiencies

Our bodies become nutrient deficient when we consume too much refined sugar. When we eat these foods, our system needs to pull nutrients from our body's stores so we can properly process the refined foods.[26]

Blood Sugar Imbalance

Refined sugars and flours get digested very quickly, leading to a rapid rise in blood-sugar levels.[27] Unstable blood sugar needs to be avoided because it can lead to symptoms such as fatigue, tiredness, jitteriness, and cravings for the wrong types of foods. Ultimately, uncontrolled blood sugar can lead to diabetes. Eradicating sugar-laden foods from our diet, and replacing them with natural, high-fibre, unrefined, and unprocessed carbohydrates will help reduce these rapid spikes in blood-sugar levels.

Obesity
Consuming too many carbohydrates like refined sugars and flours can cause obesity. Once the body has used up all the carbs it needs to provide us with the energy we require, the remainder gets converted into body fat.[28]

Increased Free-Radical Activity
Free-radical activity is happening all the time in our bodies. Free radicals are the molecules that cause damage to our body's tissues, and if they are not balanced with antioxidants, disease and illness can set in. Health concerns caused by free radicals include inflammatory problems, allergies, hyperactivity, a supressed immune system, and cardiovascular disease. Some factors that promote free radical activity include stress, environmental chemicals, food additives, and sugar.[29] Why not try to reduce the amount of free radicals in your body by reducing your intake of refined sugars and flours?

REFINED SUGAR ALTERNATIVES

Since refined white sugar offers our bodies little in terms nutritional value, and causes issues for us all, you may want to try some of these sugar alternatives the next time you reach for that sweetener or embark on a baking extravaganza!

HONEY
Honey in its raw, natural form is full of natural antioxidants, vitamins, minerals, and enzymes, including zinc, potassium, vitamin B6, and B3. Produced by our busy little friends, the bees, this sweetener is wonderful when used in baked goods, smoothies, or as a natural cold remedy.

MAPLE SYRUP

Maple syrup, made right here in Canada, contains so many beneficial nutrients, including manganese, vitamin B2, zinc, magnesium, and calcium. It's great to use in cooking, baking, or drizzled over your favourite breakfast dish. (I'm thinking pancakes again!)

COCONUT SUGAR

Coconut sugar offers a really interesting caramel flavour and is a perfect substitute for white sugar. This sugar is much lower on the glycemic index than refined white sugar. For the uninitiated, the glycemic index is a method for gauging the degree to which a given food item affects the rise in your blood sugar after eating, with a lower rating indicating a slower rate for digestion and sugar absorption, resulting in just a small rise in blood sugar, and a higher rating meaning a sharp and unwanted blood-sugar spike.[30] Coconut sugar can be used exactly as refined sugar would be used in any recipe. I love it and use it a lot!

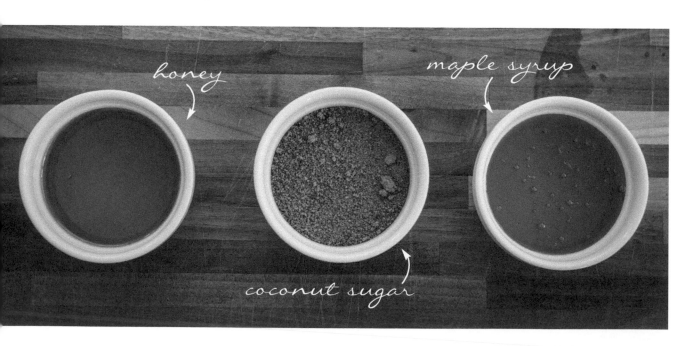

honey   maple syrup   coconut sugar

BLACKSTRAP MOLASSES

Blackstrap molasses is a by-product of the white sugar refining process. It contains all the vitamins and minerals that were absorbed by the sugar plant from the soil that doesn't make it to the nutritionally barren white sugar. These nutrients include iron, calcium, potassium, and magnesium, and the rich, sweet, distinct flavour of blackstrap molasses is a treat to use in cooking or baking recipes. Blackstrap molasses shouldn't be confused with its more processed and less beneficial cousin, fancy molasses.

STEVIA

Stevia is an herb that is much sweeter than white sugar, so only small amounts are needed. Stevia can be used when cooking or baking, and is available in liquid or powdered form.

So this concludes our quick tour of three nutritional nasties: dairy, gluten, and refined sugar. Now that we've seen the plethora of options available to replace these prevalent yet unnecessary ingredients in our everyday diets, it's time to move on to some recipes of my own creation. You'll find no dairy, zero gluten, and not one trace of refined sugar in any of these recipes, yet they all taste great! With some experimentation, I have been able to create these variations of traditional Newfoundland and Labrador favourites, along with some new, nutritionally smart ideas for using local ingredients from The Rock to craft some tasty and healthy dishes, dinners, and treats. Hope you enjoy!

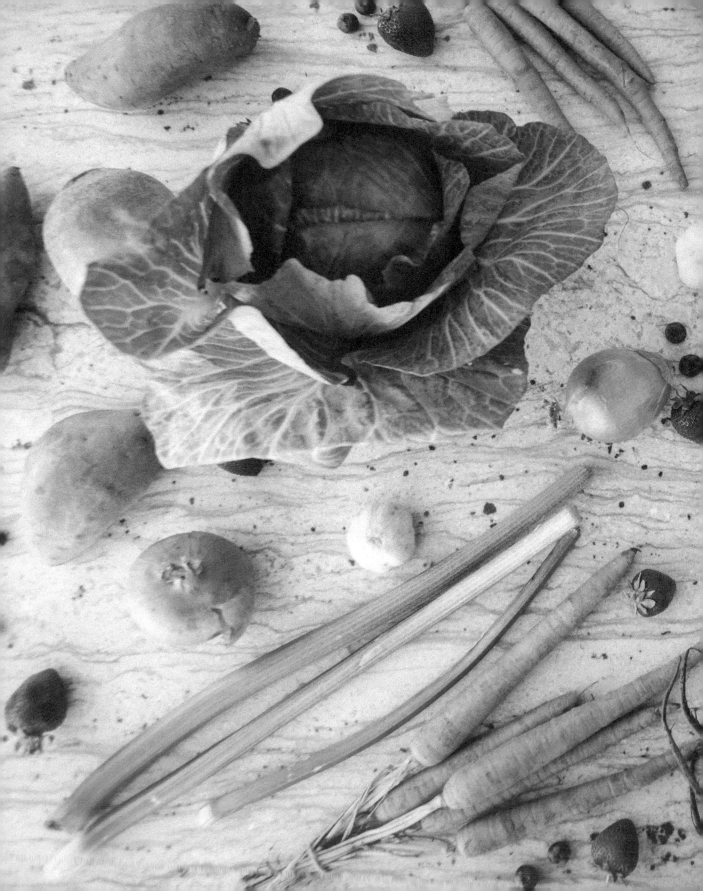

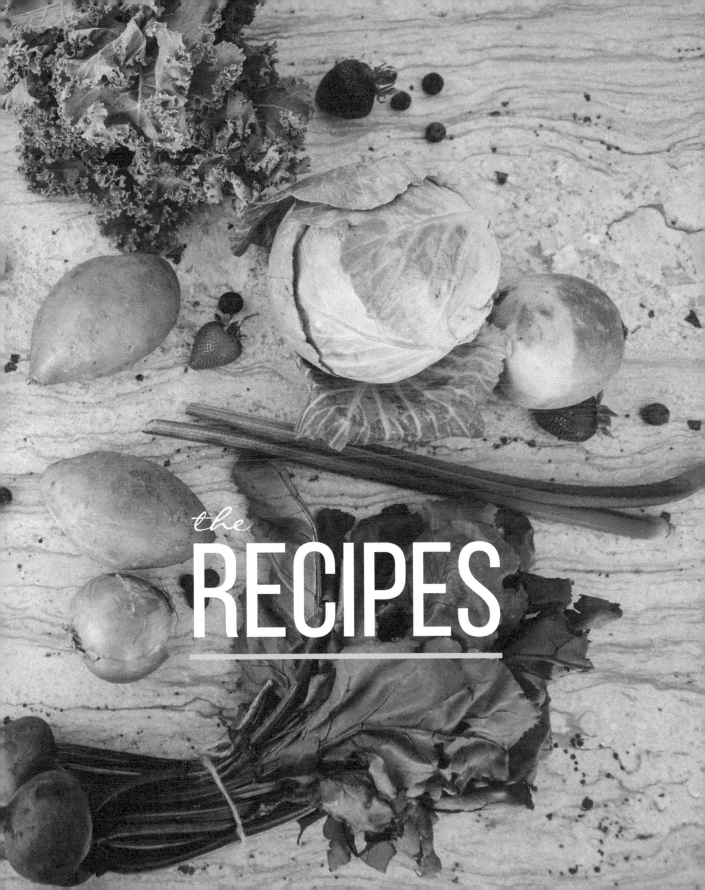

the
RECIPES

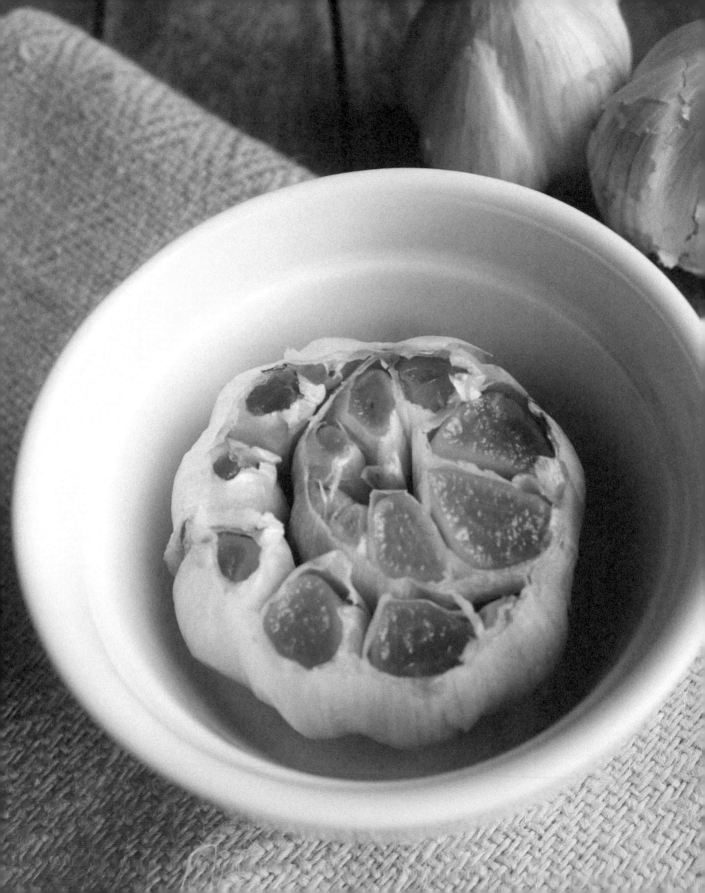

Opposite: Roasted Garlic (PAGE 49)

Condiments

TARTAR SAUCE

PREP TIME: 10 minutes

1 cup cashews,
  soaked for 6 hours or
  overnight

4 tbsp water

1 tsp dried dill

¼ tsp mustard powder

1 tsp freshly squeezed
  lemon juice

1 tsp honey

¼ tsp onion powder

2 tbsp capers, chopped

Tartar sauce is always a big hit when paired with a serving of classic battered codfish. While many mass-produced tartar sauces contain additives and/or preservatives, my homemade tartar sauce combines tasty herbs and spices and utilizes whole foods to keep it nutritious and delicious. And since tartar just ain't tartar without that trademark creaminess, cashew cream is the secret ingredient to achieve that perfect blend of taste and texture without the need for dairy.

1 Add all ingredients except the capers into a blender and blend until you reach a smooth consistency.

2 Thoroughly mix capers through cashew mixture.

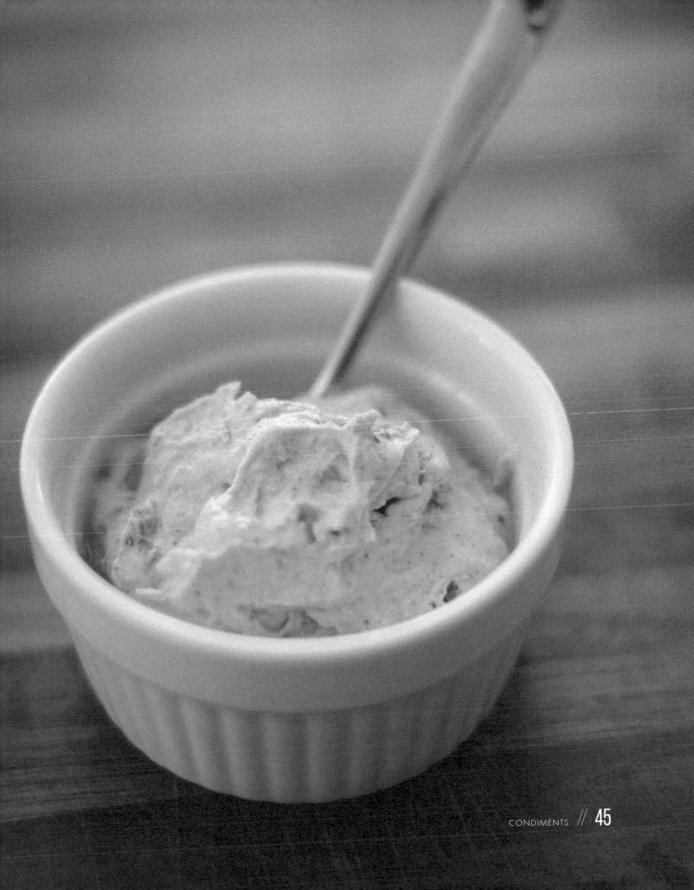

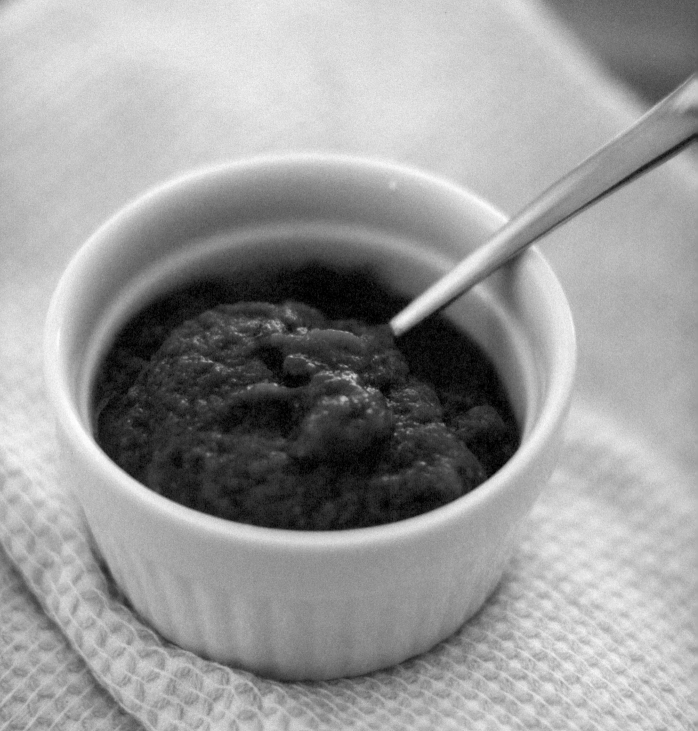

HOMEMADE KETCHUP

YIELDS 1 CUP

PREP TIME: 5 minutes

In Newfoundland, like everywhere else in North America, ketchup is one of the most common condiments on the table. Whether served with fish cakes, burgers, or a plate of fries, that familiar red bottle is never far from reach. This Homemade Ketchup ditches the scary amounts of sugar found in store-bought ketchups and achieves its tang and texture through an easy combination of wholesome ingredients.

- **1 can of organic tomato paste**
- **¼ cup apple-cider vinegar**
- **¼ cup water**
- **½ tsp sea salt**
- **½ tsp garlic powder**
- **½ tsp onion powder**
- **½ tsp parsley**
- **½ tsp mustard powder**

1 Combine all ingredients in a small bowl and mix well.

BAKEAPPLE JAM

YIELDS 1 CUP

PREP TIME: 5 minutes
COOK TIME: 10 minutes

1 cup bakeapples
1 tbsp honey
½ tbsp chia seeds

Living in a province so rich in many types of tasty berries, you can bet there are going to be preserves around. My favourite jam growing up, and still to this day, is bakeapple jam. While most jams are made with white refined sugar, I used a healthier sweetener along with some extra bonus fibre in the form of chia seeds.

1 Put the bakeapples in a small pot, on medium heat. Smash berries until broken down to a sauce-like consistency.

2 Add honey and mix through the berry mixture. Heat for approximately 5 to 10 minutes, until thickened.

3 Remove from heat and put jam in a Mason jar. Allow to cool at room temperature. Add chia seeds and stir.

4 Store in refrigerator for up to one week.

ROASTED GARLIC

YIELDS 1 BULB

PREP TIME: 5 minutes
COOK TIME: 1 hour

Oh, garlic. You truly put the *love* in *clove*. A powerhouse of health and flavour, it's a struggle for me to keep garlic out of every recipe—I just love it! When you roast your garlic, that inimitable flavour reaches whole new heights. Add it to your favourite sauce and let it do its thing.

1 garlic bulb

extra-virgin olive oil

parchment paper

cooking twine

1 Preheat oven to 350°F.

2 Cut top off garlic bulb to expose cloves.

3 Place garlic bulb on a piece of parchment paper, enough to wrap up garlic bulb.

4 Drizzle extra-virgin olive oil over garlic bulb.

5 Wrap the parchment paper up around the garlic bulb and tie at the top with cooking twine.

6 Bake for 60 minutes, until garlic is soft.

PICKLED BEETS

YIELDS 3 MASON JARS (500 ML)

PREP TIME: 15 minutes
COOK TIME: 1 hour

9 small beets, scrubbed

1 cup water

1 cup apple-cider vinegar

6 tbsp coconut sugar

Beautiful beets! These vivid purple roots are gorgeous in colour, and they don't disappoint in the taste department! Bottle them up and you can enjoy these beauties all year round. Unfortunately, the bottling process traditionally involved lots of refined sugar, which turns them from health-giving to a nutritional nasty. But not so here! When bottling my beets, I opt for coconut sugar to provide that satisfying sweet flavour, without the unwanted spike in blood sugar!

1   Add 1 inch of water to a pot and bring to a boil. Place steamer basket inside the pot and reduce heat to low. Place beets in steamer basket and cover pot. Steam beets for around 40 to 50 minutes or until beets are soft when pierced with a fork.

2   Once beets are steamed, place them in a bowl of cold water. When they are cool enough to touch, rub the peels off.

3   Slice beets and place them in Mason jars.

4   Add water, apple-cider vinegar, and coconut sugar to a pot and bring to boil. Once boiled, pour liquid over sliced beets in jars and seal with lids.

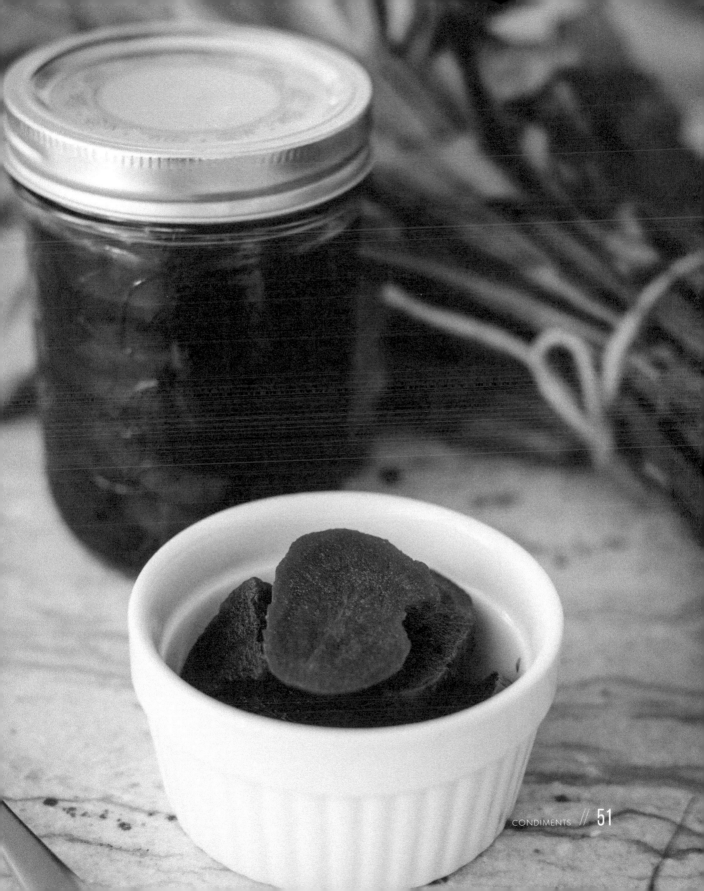

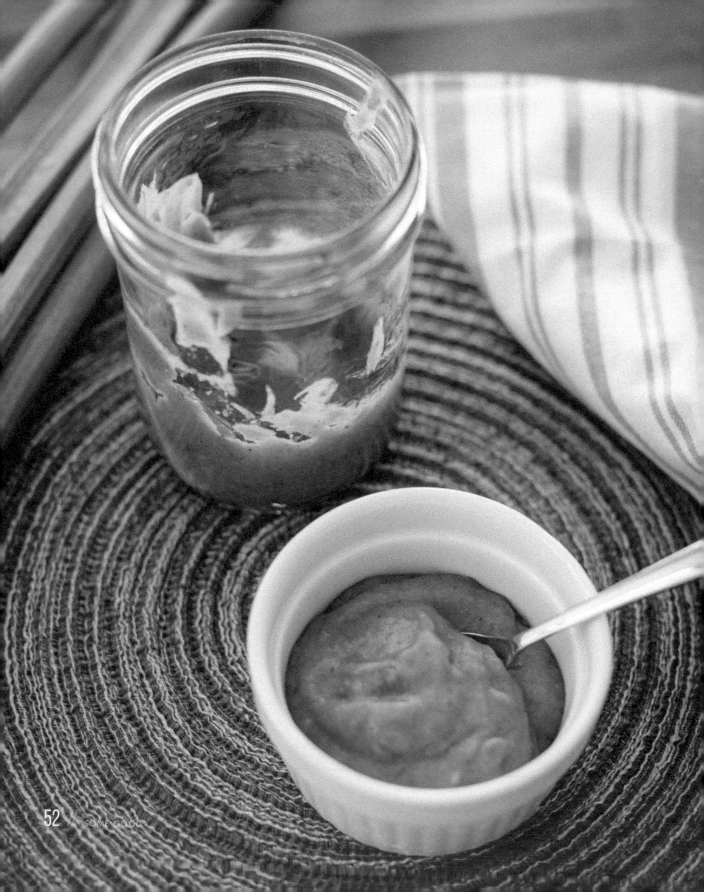

RHUBARB CHUTNEY

YIELDS ¾ CUP

PREP TIME: 10 minutes
COOK TIME: 35 minutes

What's not to love about rhubarb? Those lovely pink stalks with the signature tart taste! Rhubarb grows prevalently in Newfoundland and is a very versatile ingredient. I decided to get creative with my rhubarb and turn it into a mouth-watering chutney that makes a great addition to a nice fish dish.

1 tbsp coconut oil

½ cup finely chopped red onion

¼ cup apple-cider vinegar

½ cup honey

½ tsp ground ginger

½ tsp allspice

½ tsp sea salt

1½ cups diced rhubarb

1 Heat oil in a medium saucepan over medium heat. Cook onion until translucent, approximately 5 minutes.

2 Add apple-cider vinegar, honey, ginger, allspice, salt, and rhubarb. Bring to a boil and then let simmer for 30 minutes until mixture gets thick and rhubarb breaks down.

3 Remove from heat and let cool. Transfer mixture to a blender or food processor and combine until smooth, or leave chunky, and serve.

PARTRIDGEBERRY SALAD DRESSING

YIELDS 1 CUP

PREP TIME: 10 minutes

1 cup partridgeberries

¼ onion, chopped fine

¼ cup rice vinegar

½ cup extra-virgin olive oil

2 tsp honey

½ tsp sea salt

pinch of pepper

I love nothing more than a leafy green salad topped with an abundance of veggies, nuts, and even fruit! But nothing completes a salad quite like the perfect dressing. Most of the dressings that line the shelves of our grocery stores contain an unpronounceable horde of additives and preservatives, but making your own dressing offers the opportunity to leave these nasties on the shelf and pour on a little goodness. Did I mention that salad dressings are super easy to make?

1   Place all ingredients in a blender and blend until the mixture reaches a smooth pureed consistency.

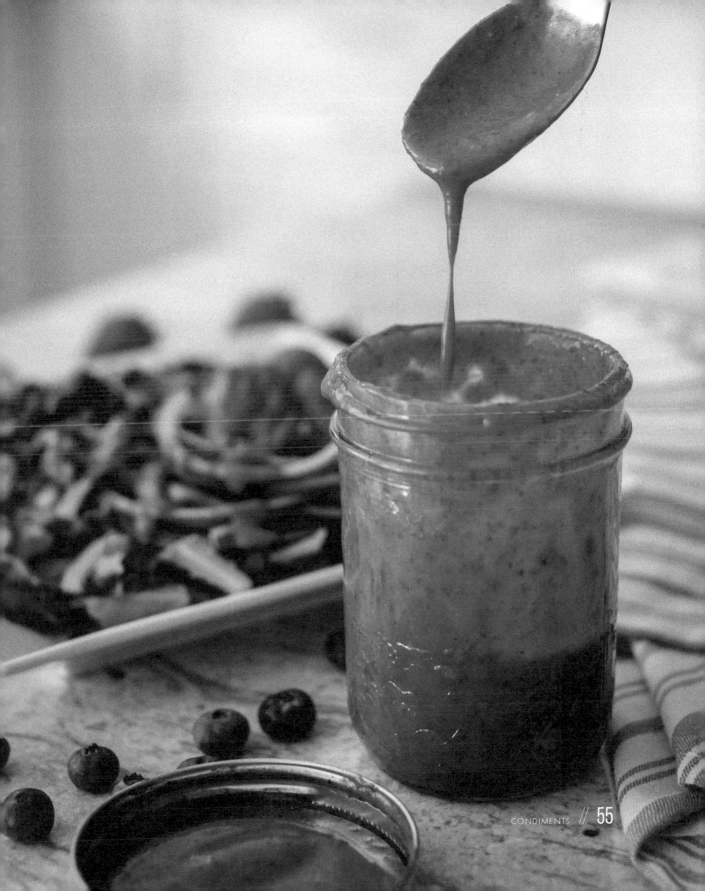

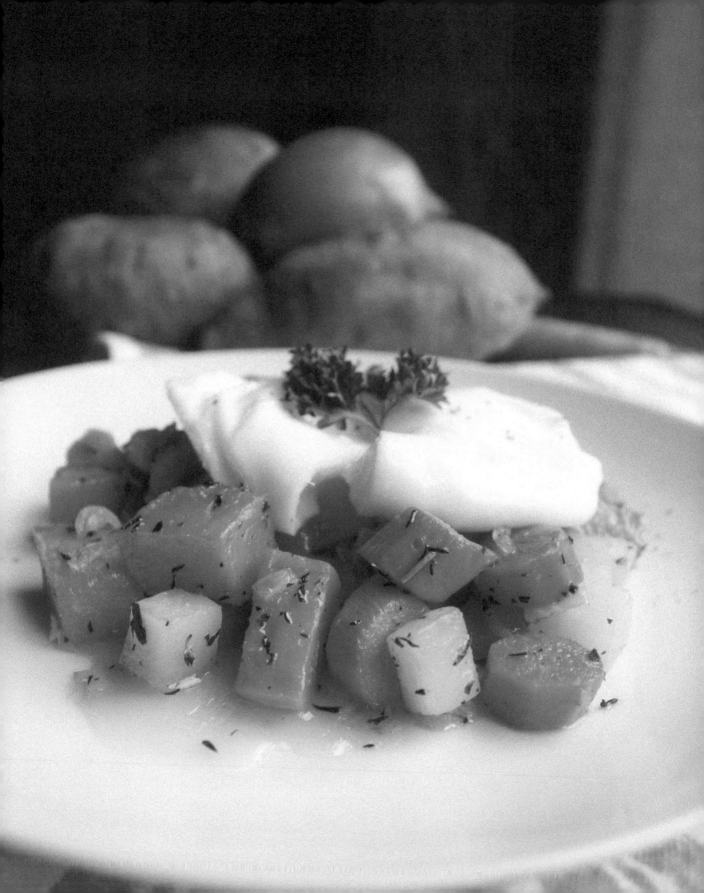

Opposite: Poached Egg on
Roasted Veg (PAGE 60)

Breakfasts

PARTRIDGEBERRY BANANA PANCAKES

YIELDS 4 SERVINGS
(2 PANCAKES EACH)

PREP TIME: 10 minutes
COOK TIME: 15 minutes

dry
INGREDIENTS

½ cup buckwheat flour

½ cup brown rice flour

2 tbsp arrowroot flour

1 tsp cinnamon

1 tsp baking powder

pinch of sea salt

wet
INGREDIENTS

1 egg

½ tbsp vanilla

**¼ cup almond milk
   or water**

additional
INGREDIENTS

¼ cup partridgeberries

½ banana, sliced

**coconut oil to grease
   pan**

Pancakes were a favourite of mine, growing up. My father wouldn't make pancakes for breakfast every day (as much as I wished he would), so it was such a treat on the occasions when he did. They still are a favourite in my house on the weekends! I've transformed my father's recipe into one that includes some very tasty Newfoundland berries and, of course, I've used gluten-free flours.

1   Combine dry ingredients in medium-sized bowl.

2   Combine wet ingredients in small bowl.

3   Pour the wet ingredients in with the dry ingredients and whisk together until combined. Fold partridgeberries and banana into mixture.

4   Grease pan over medium heat and use a ¼ cup measure to scoop out pancake mixture into the heated, greased pan.

5   When you start to see bubbles coming through the pancake mixture in the pan, flip over and cook for another minute or until golden brown.

6   Drizzle with maple syrup. Enjoy!

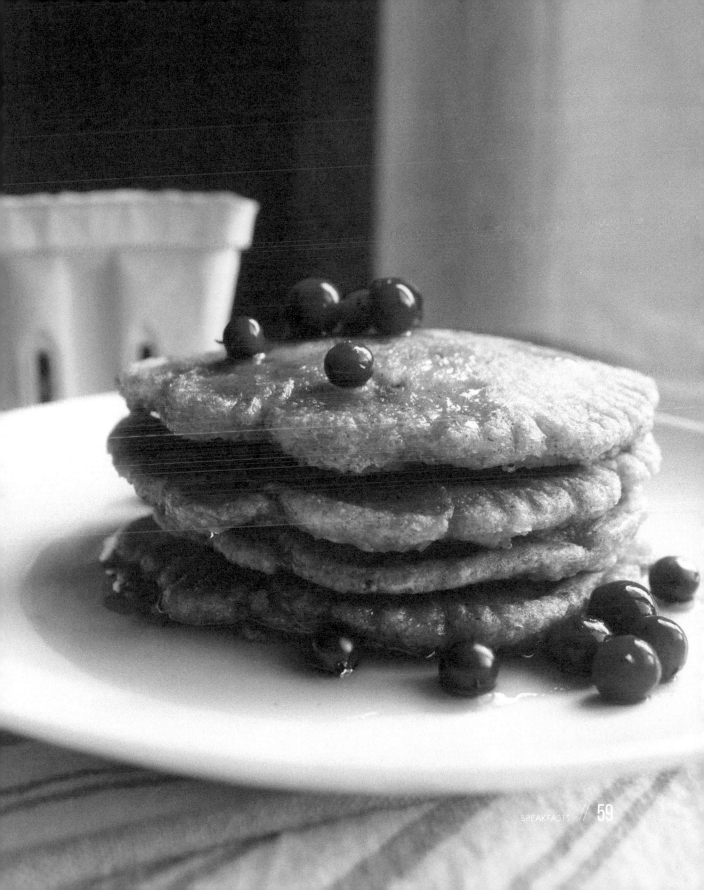

POACHED EGG *on* ROASTED VEG

Vegetables for breakfast, you may ask? Who says you can't enjoy vegetables first thing in the morning? Tradition is the only thing stopping us from starting the day with their nutrient-dense deliciousness. Newfoundland is home to an abundance of root vegetables, so it really makes sense to start your day off with a sizzling serving of roasted veggies, topped with an energy-giving poached egg. This is a great recipe if you have a little extra time in the morning. Sunday brunch, anyone?

YIELDS 2 SERVINGS

PREP TIME: 15 minutes
COOK TIME: 45 minutes

1 medium sweet potato, cubed

2 carrots, coined ¼–½ inch

½ turnip, cubed

½ onion, finely chopped

¼ tsp sea salt

dash pepper

1 tsp savoury

2 tbsp extra-virgin olive oil

2 eggs

1   Preheat oven to 375°F.

2   Place vegetables in glass baking dish and sprinkle with herbs and spices. Drizzle with oil and stir vegetables until thoroughly covered with oil, spices, and herbs.

3   Bake vegetables for 45 minutes or until vegetables are soft, stirring halfway through.

4   Bring a medium pot of water to a simmer. Crack open eggs into two separate mugs or small bowls. Stir the water to create a small whirlpool, tip the eggs into simmering water, and poach for 3 to 6 minutes. 3 minutes will give you a soft, runny yolk.

5   Remove egg from water with a slotted spoon and place on a piece of paper towel to absorb water. Plate vegetables and place the poached egg on top. Sprinkle with some extra sea salt and pepper.

PARTRIDGEBERRY PUCKER SMOOTHIE

YIELDS 2 SERVINGS
(APPROX 1 CUP EACH)

PREP TIME: 5 minutes

Pucker up, smoothie lovers! This smooth and substantial beverage offers a balance of sweet and tart tastes, all in one frosty glass. It's a cool, tasty treat packed with antioxidants thanks to those delicious Newfoundland berries—partridgeberry and blueberry. A great way to start the day or fuel you through the afternoon.

1 Combine all ingredients in a blender and blend until you reach a smooth consistency. Enjoy!

1½ cups spinach, packed loosely

½ cup frozen partridgeberries

½ cup frozen blueberries

1 banana

1 tbsp honey

2 tbsp hemp hearts

½ to 1 cup almond milk

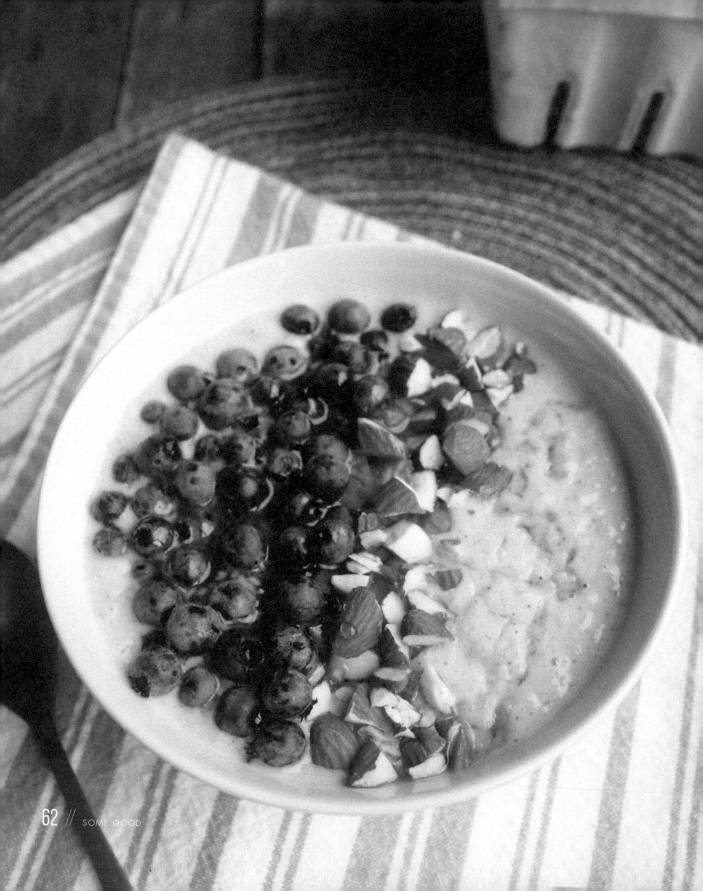

BLUEBERRY OATMEAL BOWL

YIELDS 1 SERVING

PREP TIME: 5 minutes
COOK TIME: 10 minutes

Oatmeal reminds me of my grandmother. I have fond memories of her preparing oatmeal for my grandfather and I on cold winter days while we warmed ourselves by the woodstove. Oatmeal consistency is a very personal matter. I prefer mine not too thick, not to thin, but just right. My grandfather, on the other hand, insisted on having his very thin—almost like soup. By adjusting the amount of almond milk In this recipe, you can dial the thickness up or down. Whether you're for thick, thin, or *just right*, this Blueberry Oatmeal Bowl is sure to warm your soul.

- 1 cup water
- ½ cup gluten-free quick rolled oats
- ¼ tsp cinnamon
- ¼ cup almond milk
- ¼ cup fresh blueberries
- 2 tbsp almonds, chopped
- 1 tbsp maple syrup (optional)

1 Bring water to a boil in a medium-sized sauce pan.

2 Add oats and cinnamon and reduce heat to simmer. Cook oats until you reach a thick consistency, around 3-5 minutes.

3 Stir in almond milk until it becomes warm and you reach desired consistency of oatmeal, around 3-5 minutes.

4 Pour oatmeal in bowl and top with blueberries and almonds. You can drizzle with maple syrup for extra sweetness.

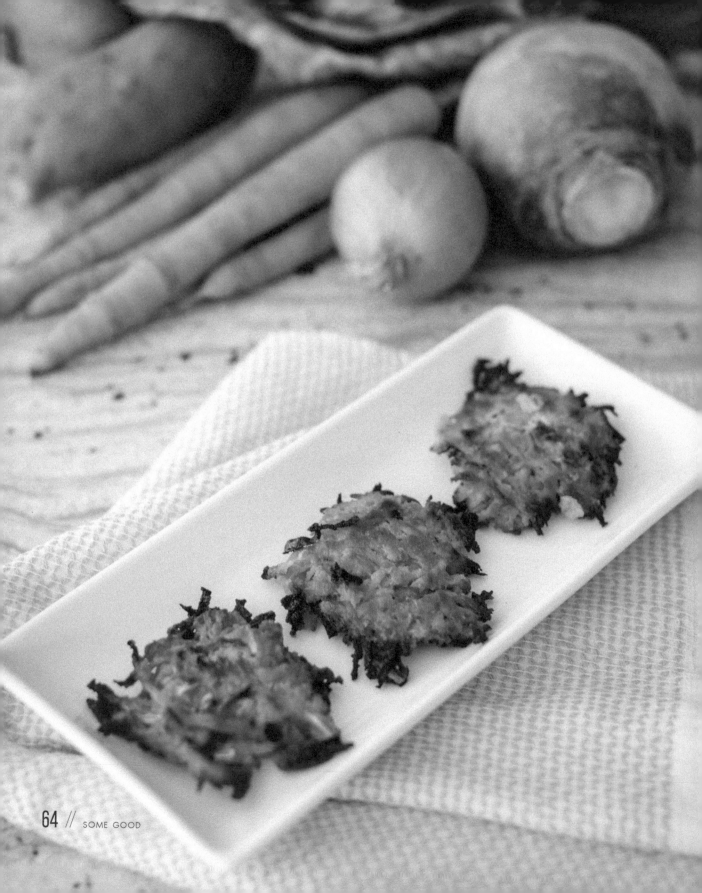

Opposite: Jiggs Dinner Veggie Cakes (PAGE 74)

Appetizers

PAN-SEARED SCALLOPS *with* CASHEW CREAM ROASTED GARLIC SAUCE

Newfoundland is awash with a diverse seafood bounty. Not only do the well-known codfish call our coast home, but scallops are also present in abundance. There are few seafood treats tastier than pan-fried scallops. Smother these little dollops of deliciousness in my dairy-free Cashew Cream Roasted Garlic Sauce and you have a very flavourful—and nutritious—dish!

YIELDS 10 SCALLOPS

PREP TIME: 10 minutes
COOK TIME: 8 minutes

½ cup water

1 cup cashews,
   soaked for 2 hours or overnight

¼ tsp sea salt

1 tsp savoury

4 cloves roasted garlic *(recipe on page 49)*

10 scallops

1 tbsp extra-virgin olive oil

dash sea salt

dash pepper

1 **MAKE THE SAUCE:** Add water, cashews, ¼ teaspoon sea salt, savoury, and roasted garlic to blender and blend until you get a smooth consistency. Set aside.

2 Heat oil in pan over medium heat. Add scallops and heat for 2 minutes. Sprinkle with a dash of sea salt and pepper. Flip scallops and heat for another 2-3 minutes or until scallops are cooked through.

3 You can remove scallops from heat and serve with desired amount of unwarmed sauce, or you can take desired amount of sauce and add to pan with scallops and warm for about 1 minute. If there is sauce left over, store in refrigerator up to 3-4 days.

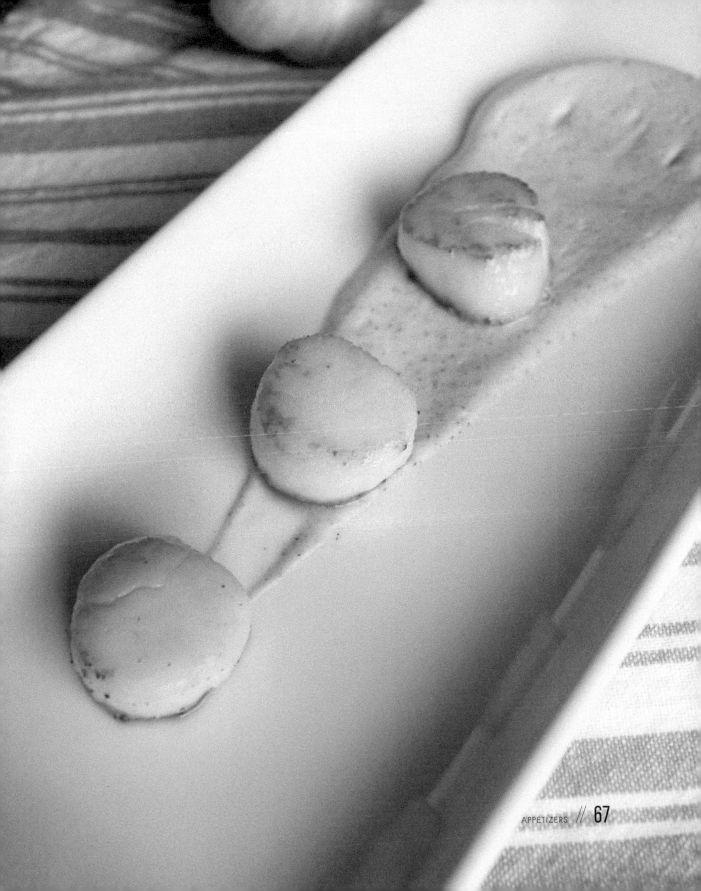

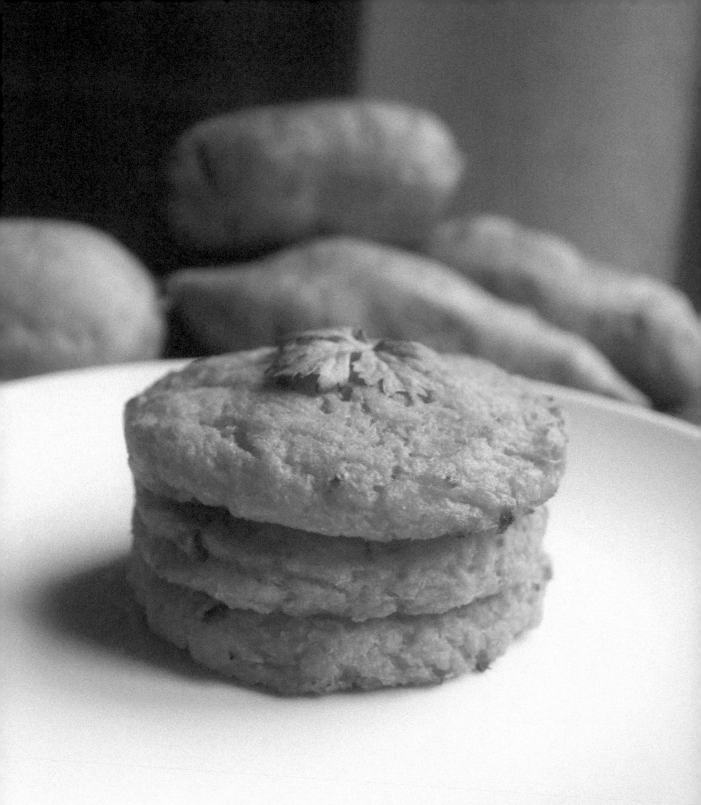

SWEET POTATO CAKES

My grandmother is the master of potato cakes—a Newfoundland staple and a favourite of our family. While Nan made them the traditional way, using white potato, I decided to see what it would be like to make them with sweet potato, to amp up the nutrient profile. Turns out, these Sweet Potato Cakes taste great and provide a healthier twist on the original dish.

1 Place sweet potatoes in a steam basket and steam for 20 minutes or until tender.

2 Once steamed remove steam basket from pot, set aside, and let cool for 10-12 minutes.

3 Preheat oven to 350°F and place parchment paper on large baking sheet.

4 When cooled, place sweet potatoes in bowl and mash. Add brown rice flour and thoroughly combine.

5 Use a ¼ cup to measure out potato mixture and use hands to form into round cakes and place on baking sheet.

6 Use a pastry or basting brush and brush coconut oil on the top of cakes and bake for 30 minutes.

7 Once cooked turn on broiler for 4-5 minutes until tops are slightly browned.

YIELDS 8 CAKES

PREP TIME: 15 minutes
COOK TIME: 55 minutes

3 medium potatoes, peeled and diced

6 tbsp brown rice flour

1 tbsp coconut oil, melted

LOBSTER STUFFED MUSHROOMS

Lobster has gained a reputation as one of the finest 'feeds' from the sea. Every summer, these incredible crustaceans are caught in Newfoundland waters and widely available in our stores. A firm favourite of seafood connoisseurs, lobster tastes great all on its own. Upon boiling in water, it is often cracked open, the succulent flesh retrieved and dipped in butter. But when you stuff that delicious meat into a mushroom with my creamy, herbed filling, it makes for a taste so sensational, you'll hardly believe it's actually really good for you!

YIELDS 18 STUFFED MUSHROOMS

PREP TIME: 15 minutes
COOK TIME: 22 minutes

1 cup cashews, soaked overnight

4 tbsp water

¼ tsp sea salt

1 tsp thyme

½ tsp garlic powder

1¼ cup finely chopped lobster

18 cremini mushrooms,
   washed and stems removed

almond flour

extra-virgin olive oil

1 Preheat oven to 400°F.

2 Combine cashews, water, salt, thyme, and garlic powder in a blender and blend until you reach a smooth consistency.

3 Remove from blender and place in a bowl. Add lobster and mix thoroughly.

4 Place mushrooms on baking sheet and stuff mushrooms with lobster mixture. Sprinkle with almond flour and drizzle with oil.

5 Place in oven and bake for 20 minutes. After 20 minutes, broil for 2 minutes or until golden brown on top.

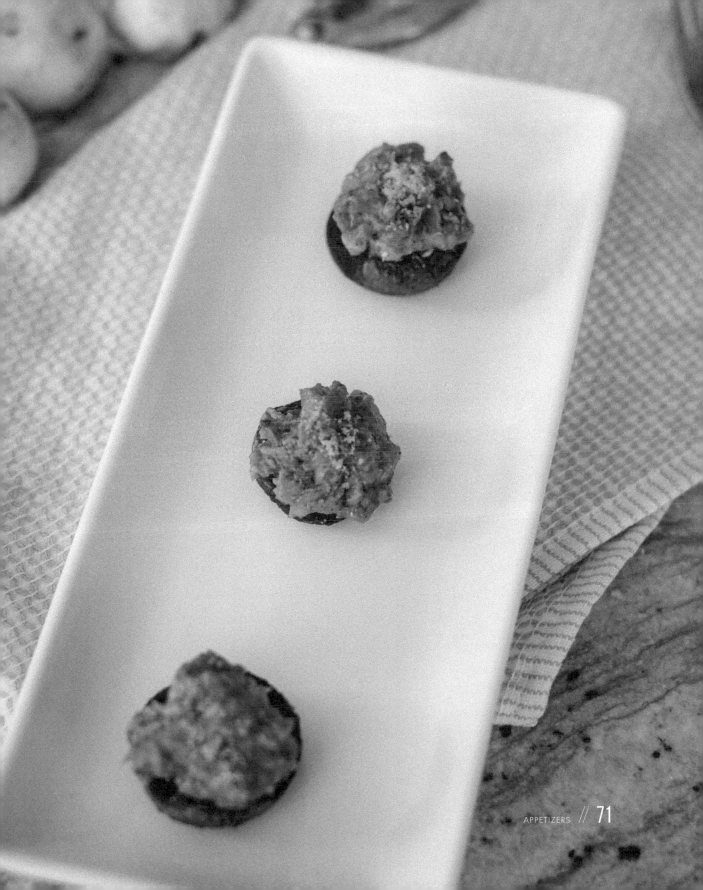

CAULIFLOWER COD CAKES

Fish cakes are an absolute favourite of mine and have been since I was a kid. They are always on my list of 'must makes' when I visit my mom, typically served with a generous side of baked beans—a match made in heaven! In order to up the healthy, I created a fishcake with a cauliflower rather than a white potato base. I think you'll be impressed with the results!

YIELDS 12 PATTIES

PREP TIME: 25 minutes
COOK TIME: 15 minutes

2 cups cauliflower rice
   (approximately ½ head)

1½ lbs cod

1 tsp sea salt

dash black pepper

1 tbsp savoury

½ small onion, chopped finely

1 large egg

½ cup almond flour

extra-virgin olive oil for cooking
   in pan

1   **MAKE THE CAULIFLOWER RICE:** Chop ½ cauliflower into florets and place in a food processor. Pulse until you reach a rice texture.

2   Add 1 tablespoon of extra-virgin olive oil to a medium heated pan. Add cauliflower rice to pan and cook for about 5-8 minutes, stirring occasionally until cauliflower becomes tender and fragrant. Once cooked, set aside to cool.

3   Add 1 tablespoon of extra-virgin olive oil to a medium heated pan. Place cod in pan and sprinkle with ¼ teaspoon of sea salt and a dash of pepper. Cook for 4 minutes and then flip and cook on the other side for 4 minutes or until the fish is cooked through. Sprinkle with ¼ teaspoon sea salt and a dash of pepper. Once cooked, set aside and let cool.

4 Place cauliflower rice, ½ teaspoon sea salt, dash of pepper, savoury, onion, egg, and almond flour in a bowl. Next add cod and thoroughly combine.

5 Add 1 tablespoon of oil in a medium heated pan. Use a ¼ cup measure to make fish cakes. Use hands to firmly pack the cake mould together and place in pan.

6 Cook each fish cake for 3-5 minutes or until golden brown and then flip to brown the other side. Continue doing this until all fish cakes are made, adding extra oil to the pan when needed.

tip // *If you like a condiment with your fish cakes, try coupling them with the Tartar Sauce or Homemade Ketchup in this cookbook!*

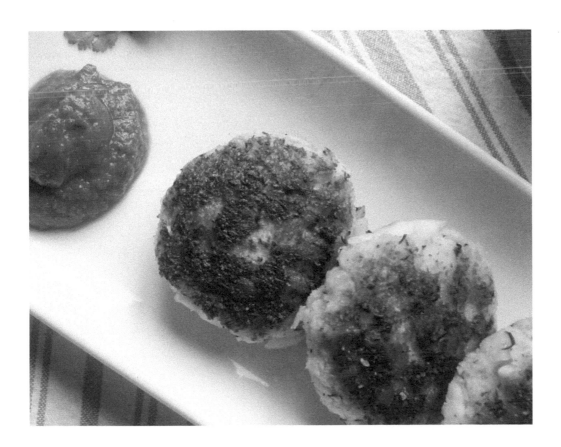

JIGGS DINNER VEGGIE CAKES

Ah, Jiggs Dinner. Perhaps Newfoundland's most famous dish. This recipe takes inspiration from the classic home-cooked meal, utilizing the vegetables found in a traditional Newfoundland Jiggs Dinner: potato, carrot, turnip, and cabbage. While Jiggs Dinner always makes for a tasty feed, the boiling involved has the unfortunate side effect of sapping nutrients from the veggies. Baking these vegetables, all together in a delicious veggie cake, gives Jiggs Dinner a new life and an enhanced nutrient profile!

YIELDS 12 CAKES

PREP TIME: 25 minutes
COOK TIME: 35 minutes

1 cup grated sweet potato

1 cup grated carrot

1 cup grated turnip

1 cup finely chopped cabbage

½ small onion, chopped finely

1 egg

½ tsp sea salt

½ cup brown rice flour

1 tsp baking powder

¼ cup extra-virgin olive oil

1 Preheat oven to 350°F and line baking sheet with parchment paper.

2 Mix potato, carrot, turnip, cabbage, and onion in a medium bowl.

3 Add egg and combine in vegetable mixture.

4 Add salt, flour, and baking powder and mix thoroughly through vegetable and egg mixture.

5 Use a ¼ cup measure to scoop out cake mixture, and place on baking sheet lined with parchment paper. Continue to do this until all the mixture is gone.

6 Drizzle extra-virgin olive oil over the cakes and bake for 25 minutes. At 25 minutes, flip the cakes over and bake for another 10 minutes.

PEA SUPER SOUP

Pea soup is such a warming, wholesome soup to enjoy on a cold day. It is a Newfoundland favourite and definitely a favourite of mine. My interpretation of pea soup is just as satisfying, with some extra nutritional benefits. With the addition of the lovely spice, turmeric, and the removal of ham/salt beef, this soup becomes super nourishing and delicious! Finish it off with my gluten-free Pea Super Soup Dumplings, included in the Breads section of this cookbook.

1 Place water, peas, sea salt, pepper, and turmeric in a pot and bring to a boil. Once reaching boiling point, reduce to simmer.

2 Simmer peas and spices for 1 hour and 30 minutes or until peas are almost cooked. Stir occasionally so peas do not burn onto pot.

3 Add vegetables and cook soup for another 30 minutes, stirring occasionally.

4 IF MAKING DUMPLINGS: Drop dumpling batter onto soup during the last 15 minutes of cook time and cover. Refer to Pea Super Soup Dumplings (page 126) for the recipe.

YIELDS 6 SERVINGS

PREP TIME: 15 minutes
COOK TIME: 2 hours

10 cups water

2 cups yellow split peas

1 tsp sea salt

½ tsp pepper

1 tsp turmeric

1¼ cup coined carrots (approximately 3 carrots)

¾ cup diced turnip (approximately ½ small turnip)

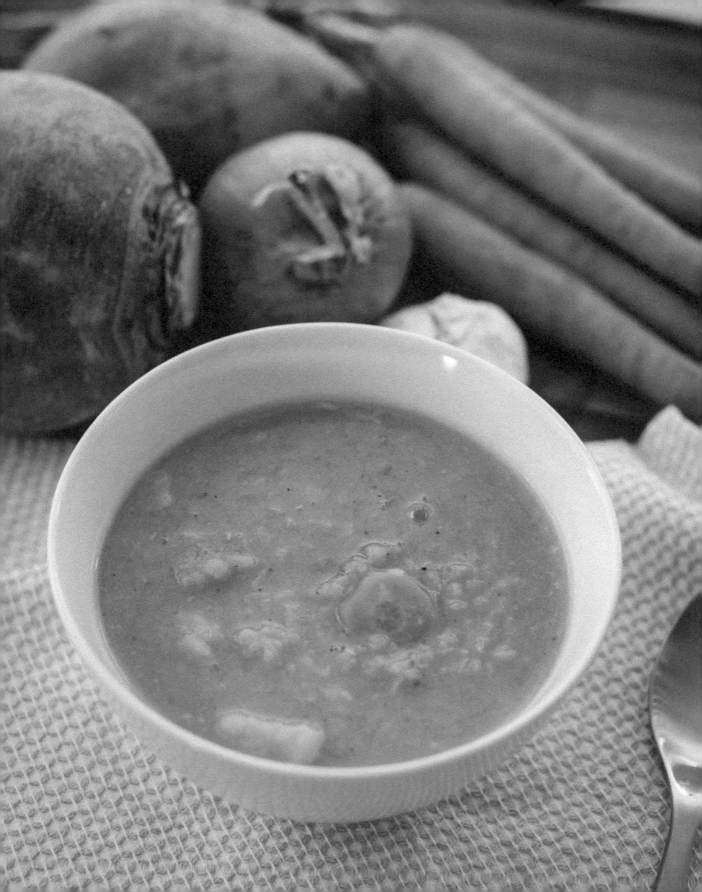

Opposite: Curry Lentil Root Stew (PAGE 91)

Mains

SEAFOOD CHOWDER

YIELDS 6 SERVINGS

PREP TIME: 30 minutes
COOK TIME: 45 minutes

2 tbsp coconut oil, plus 2 tbsp

2 cloves garlic, minced

½ yellow onion, chopped finely

1 head cauliflower, chopped

4 cups water, plus 8 tbsp,
  plus ¼ cup

1 cup cashews, soaked for
  6 hours or overnight

¼ cup sliced celery

½ cup coined carrot

½ cup chopped small sweet
  potato

4 scallops, cut into quarters

12 small shrimp, cooked

½ fillet cod, cut into 1-inch
  cubes

½ small fillet salmon, skinned
  and cut into 1-inch cubes

1 tsp savoury

½ tsp sea salt

¼ tsp pepper

There are two places you are pretty much guaranteed to find seafood chowder: Any Newfoundland tourist restaurant, and my parents' home on Christmas Eve! Creamy, warming, and delicious, there's so much to appreciate in a bowl of chowder. I just love the flavours the different seafoods provide, but the dairy I can do without. This Seafood Chowder is just as creamy and delicious as your favourite restaurant or homemade chowder, but without the dairy. Don't believe me? Give it a try!

1 Melt 2 tablespoons of oil in a large pot over medium heat. Add onion and garlic and cook until onions are translucent.

2 Next, add cauliflower and 4 cups of water. Bring to a boil and simmer for 12 minutes.

3 While cauliflower is cooking, add the soaked cashews and 8 tablespoons of water to a blender and blend until smooth.

4 When cauliflower is cooked, transfer your cauliflower, onion, and garlic to a vented food processor or blender. Blend until you reach a smooth consistency. Set aside.

5 In a large pot, melt 2 tablespoons of oil and sauté the scallops, cod, and salmon for about 5 minutes until fish is almost cooked. Then add shrimp, ¼ cup water, celery, carrot, sweet potato, and cashew cream mixture. Cook for another 2 minutes.

6 Then add cauliflower mixture, savoury, salt, and pepper.

7 Simmer for 20 minutes until vegetables are cooked, stirring occasionally to prevent the chowder from burning on the bottom of the pot.

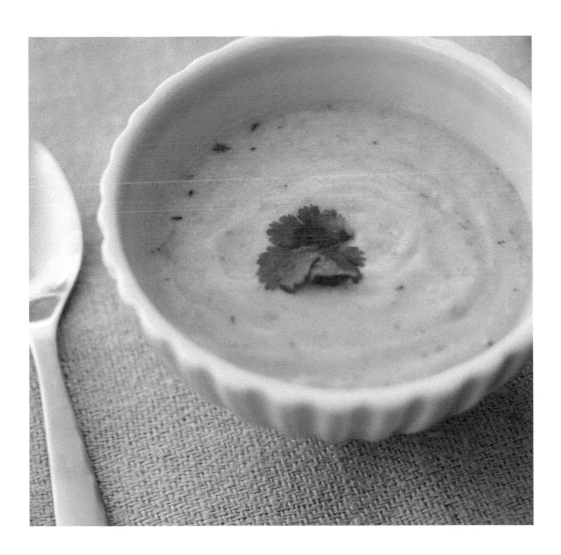

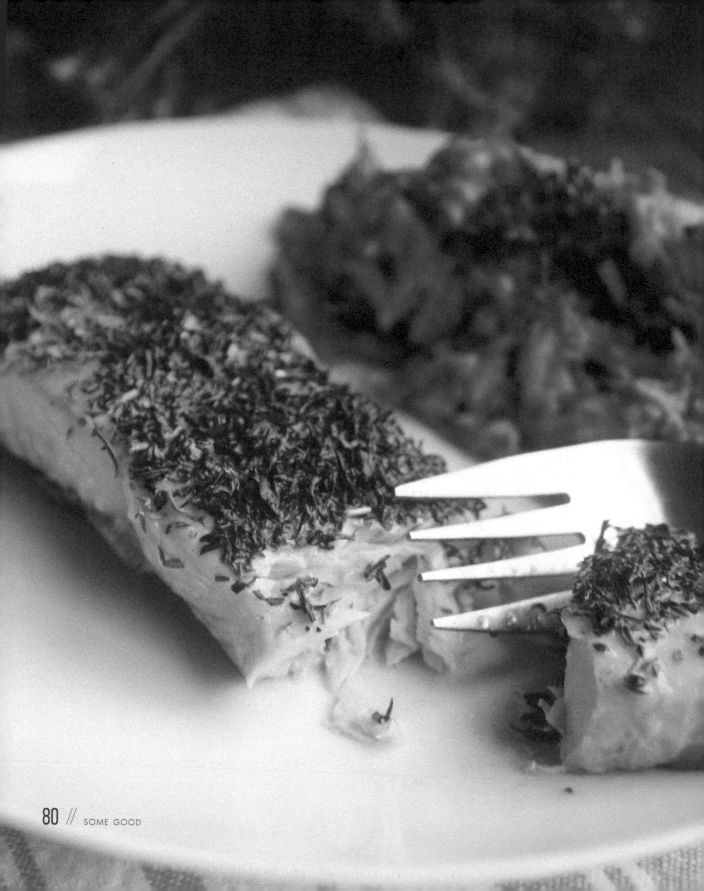

SAVOURY SALMON

YIELDS 2 SERVINGS

PREP TIME: 5 minutes
COOK TIME: 15 minutes

My father loves to go salmon fishing. He'll put on his waders, head out into the rushing water, and wait patiently for his catch. Fortunately for the rest of us, he's a good fisher and always brings home a wild salmon for us to enjoy! Salmon makes for a great main, or a welcome addition to any spread with its distinctive flavour. It also provides us with some healthy fats. When you pair salmon with one of Newfoundland's favourite herbs—savoury—you get a truly satisfying fish dish.

2 salmon filets

dash sea salt

dash pepper

2 tsp savoury

2 tbsp extra-virgin olive oil

1   Preheat oven to 375°F.

2   Place salmon fillets on baking sheet. Sprinkle salmon with sea salt, pepper, and savoury. Drizzle with oil.

3   Place in oven and bake for 15 minutes or until the salmon is cooked through and flakes apart with a fork.

LENTIL CABBAGE ROLLS

YIELDS 8 CABBAGE ROLLS

PREP TIME: 45 minutes
COOK TIME: 1 hour 30 minutes

1 large cabbage

2 cups cooked green lentils

1 cup cooked brown rice

1 cup sliced mushrooms

1 onion, chopped finely

2 cloves garlic, minced

2 tsp dried parsley

½ tsp sea salt

¼ tsp cumin

739 ml organic tomato sauce

Often, cabbage rolls are made with ground meat, but I thought, why not fill them with some lentils to make them vegetarian? The result was a truly tasty twist on a traditional dish. Simply by changing up some of the ingredients we use to make our favourite dishes, we can make things healthier and just as delicious. And don't forget—protein doesn't just come from meat. The lentils in this dish are protein-packed.

1 Preheat oven to 350°F.

2 Fill a large pot with enough water to cover cabbage, and bring to a boil.

3 Remove all ragged outer leaves and remove as much of the core of the cabbage as possible without cutting up the rest of the cabbage.

4 Place cabbage in the pot, core-end up. Remove each of its leaves using kitchen tongs as they soften and become loose. Make sure you have 8 leaves for your rolls.

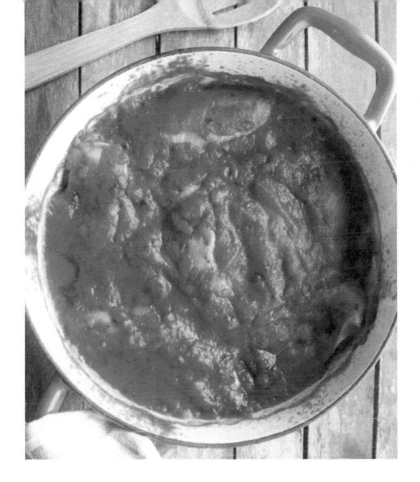

5 Rinse cabbage leaves under cold water so they are cool enough to handle.

6 In a medium bowl, mix the lentils, rice, mushrooms, onion, garlic, parsley, salt, and cumin until thoroughly combined.

7 Pour half of the tomato sauce in the bottom of a Dutch oven.

8 Take one cabbage leaf at a time and cut off the top part of the leaf where the stem is thick, just about an inch. Take ⅓ cup of filling, place in the centre of the cabbage leaf, and roll the cabbage leaf, keeping the sides tucked in. Place cabbage roll in Dutch oven. Continue to do this until all 8 leaves are filled and placed in the Dutch oven.

9 Take the remainder of the tomato sauce and pour over the cabbage rolls, spreading evenly, covering all the rolls.

10 Place in oven and bake for 1 hour and 30 minutes.

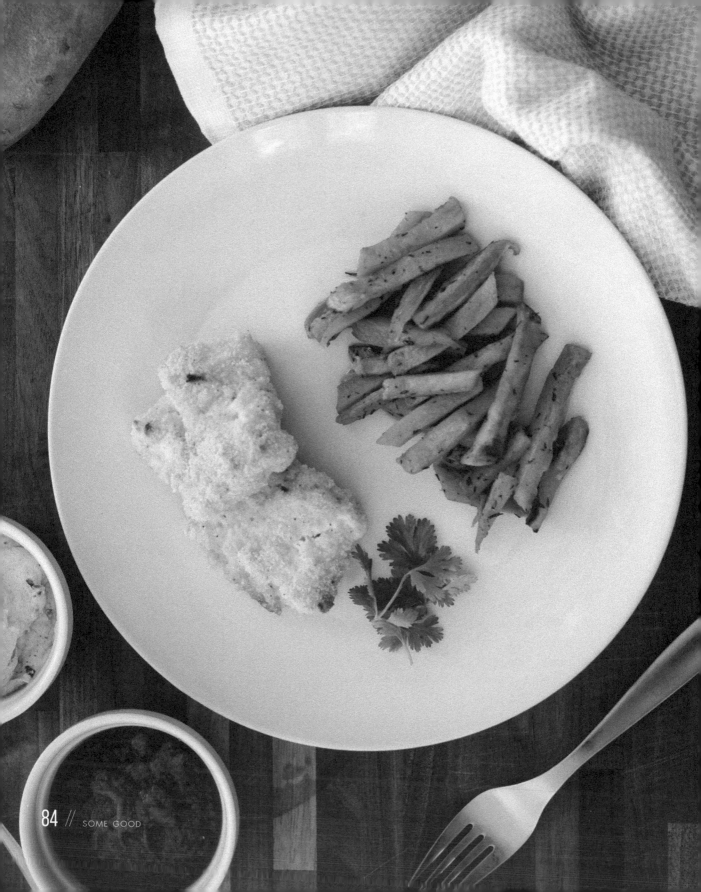

BATTERED BAKED COD

YIELDS 2 SERVINGS

PREP TIME: 15 minutes
COOK TIME: 24 minutes

When you think of the most common Newfoundland dishes, Fish and Chips will never be far from the top of the list. This time-tested pairing is as popular with locals as it is with visiting tourists, and undoubtedly delicious. What does one do when faced with the task of reimagining such an engrained staple? I wanted to maintain the taste and texture as much as possible, but without deep-frying, which unfortunately soaks the fish with rancid fats. This Battered Baked Cod still has that trademark crispy batter, with none of those nasty fats, and adds a one-two punch of hardy fibre and homemade flavour!

2 cod fillets, cut into large pieces

¼ cup brown rice flour

1 egg

½ cup almond flour

½ tsp sea salt

pinch of pepper

2 tbsp extra-virgin olive oil

1 Preheat oven to 375°F.

2 Pat dry fish with paper towel.

3 Sprinkle brown rice flour on a small plate, whisk egg in a bowl, and sprinkle almond flour on a separate plate.

4 Thoroughly combine salt and pepper with almond flour.

5 Roll fish in brown rice flour, dip into egg, and then into almond flour.

6 Place fish in baking dish and drizzle with oil.

7 Bake in the oven for 20 minutes. After 20 minutes, broil the fish for 4 minutes or until golden brown.

GARLIC SAVOURY ROAST CHICKEN

Roast chicken or turkey is always a hit in Newfoundland homes and is generally the star dish in what we call a 'Sunday Dinner'. The downside, for anyone trying to eliminate gluten, is that the bird is often filled with a dressing made with bread. To get away from the gluten, but maintain that amazing flavour, stuff your chicken or turkey with just the herbs and spices, and hold off on the bread. Served with roast veggies, the succulent taste and texture will be so satisfying, you won't miss that inflammatory dressing.

YIELDS 1 ROAST CHICKEN
(4 SERVINGS)

PREP TIME: 15 minutes
COOK TIME: 1 hour 30 minutes

1 (2½ – 3 lbs) whole chicken

½ tsp sea salt

2 tsp dried savoury

1 bulb of garlic, peel removed

1 small onion, diced

water

1 Preheat oven to 425°F.

2 Rinse chicken under cold water, pat dry with paper towel, and place in roaster.

3 Sprinkle half the salt and savoury inside the chicken and half on top of the chicken.

4 Place half the onion inside the chicken along with the full bulb of garlic.

5 Place the remainder of the onion in the bottom of the roaster, around the chicken.

6 Pour water into the roaster until there is about an inch of water from the bottom.

7 Place the chicken in the oven for 1 hour and 15 minutes, basting halfway through.

8 After 1 hour and 15 minutes, remove lid from roaster, baste one last time, and bake uncovered for another 15 minutes.

9 Remove from oven and place on platter dish to serve.

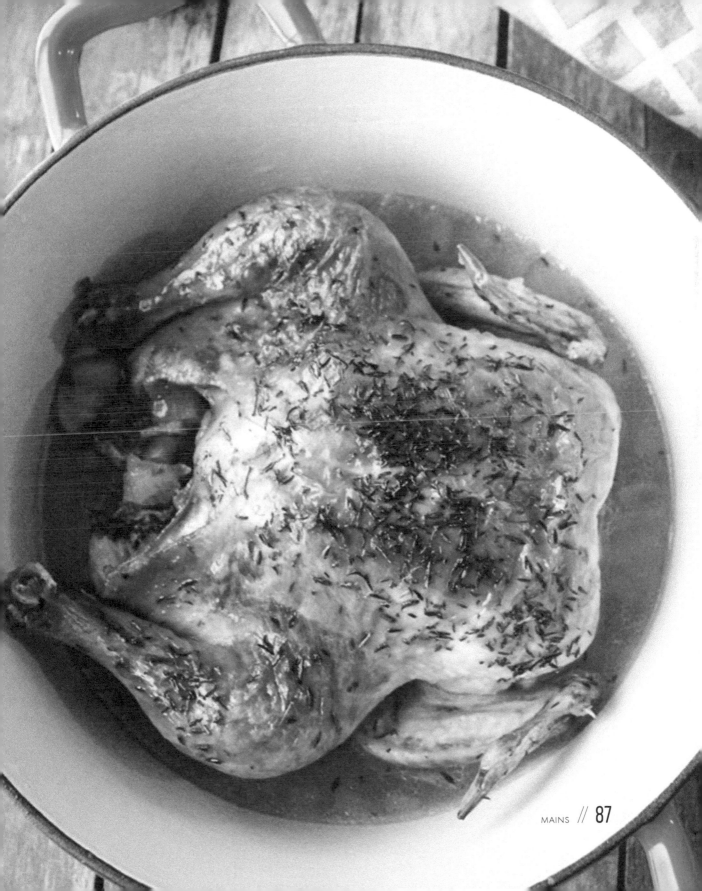

MOOSE STEW

YIELDS 5 SERVINGS

PREP TIME: 30 minutes
COOK TIME: 2½ hours

2 tbsp coconut oil

2 lbs moose meat, cut
　　into small cubes

1 onion, chopped

1 tsp garlic powder

½ tsp sea salt

¼ tsp pepper

1 tsp thyme

5 cups water, plus ¾ cup
　　water

1 cup diced carrot

1 cup diced turnip

1 cup diced sweet potato

¼ cup sliced celery

6 tbsp arrowroot flour

My father and grandfather are true Newfoundland outdoorsmen and have often hunted moose over the years, as have many Newfoundlanders. Moose will always remind me of Nan and Pop's visits, when she would stay home and hang out with the girls of the house while Pop and Dad went out hunting. Moose are such large animals, the meat from just one moose can provide families with a source of delicious meat all year round. The wild taste of moose offers a wealth of flavour to a stew, and because it's wild, it's free of the antibiotics and hormones that may be found in a farm-raised animal. Wholesome, warming, and flavourful, moose stew is a delicious treat, especially on a cold winter's day.

1　Preheat oven to 325°F.

2　Heat oil on medium to high in a cast-iron Dutch oven or frying pan.

3　Sauté moose meat, onion, and spices until moose meat becomes browned and onions become translucent, approximately 10 minutes.

4　Add 5 cups of water to the Dutch oven, or transfer moose meat mixture to a roaster and add water. Transfer Dutch oven or roaster to oven and cook for 1 hour and 30 minutes.

5 After meat has been cooking for 1 hour and 30 minutes, add vegetables to Dutch oven or roaster and return to the oven for another hour.

6 Once vegetables are tender and stew is cooked, remove from oven.

7 In a glass or Mason jar, add arrowroot flour and ¾ cup water. Stir until arrowroot flour dissolves. Add arrowroot mixture to stew and stir until completely combined and stew has thickened.

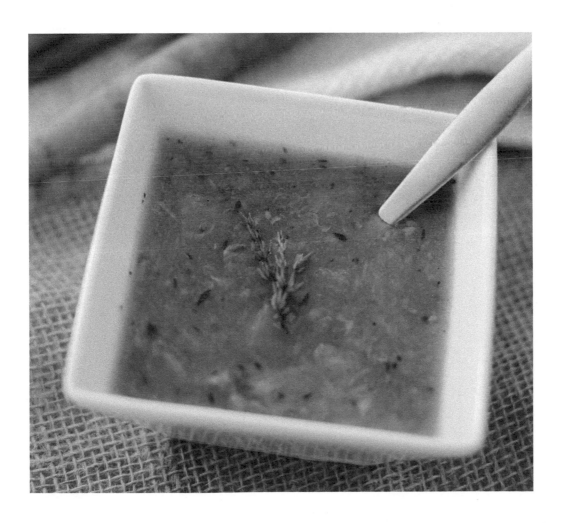

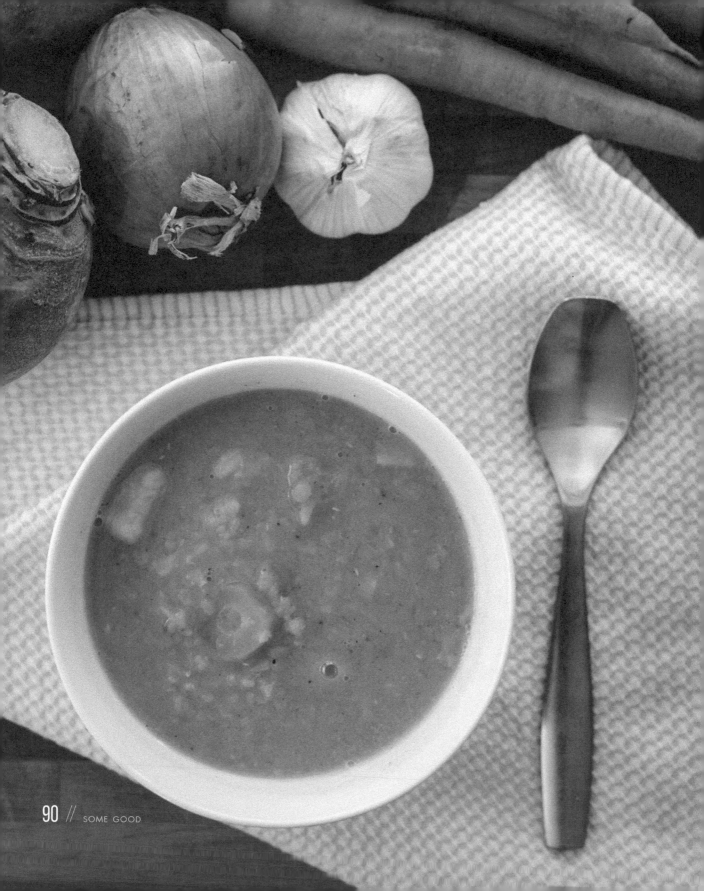

CURRY LENTIL ROOT STEW

YIELDS 4 SERVINGS

PREP TIME: 15 minutes
COOK TIME: 1 hour

We are blessed to have access to an abundance of root vegetables in Newfoundland, and we tend to eat them often! While we make good use of our roots, the ways we cook them and incorporate them tends to be pretty samey. It's always nice to take the whole ingredients you have readily available and experiment a little! I wanted to take those common root vegetables and infuse them with some non-traditional ingredients to come up with a new dish with a different flavour. This Curry Lentil Root Stew is brought to you by the abundance of roots found in Newfoundland, and the always-satisfying wonder of culinary creativity!

2 tbsp extra-virgin olive oil

1 onion, diced

1 tsp sea salt

3 cloves of garlic, minced

5 cups water

1 tsp curry powder

½ tsp turmeric

1 cup rinsed red lentils

3 carrots, coined

1 sweet potato, diced

½ turnip, diced

½ tsp pepper

1 Heat oil in large pot over medium heat. Add onion and ½ teaspoon of salt, and cook until onions become translucent, around 10 minutes.

2 Add garlic, ¼ cup of water, curry powder, and turmeric. Cook for 1 minute.

3 Stir in lentils and the remaining 4¾ cups of water, and bring to boil. Reduce heat and simmer for 20 minutes.

4 Add carrots, sweet potato, turnip, remaining ½ teaspoon of salt, and pepper. Simmer for another 30 minutes or until vegetables are tender.

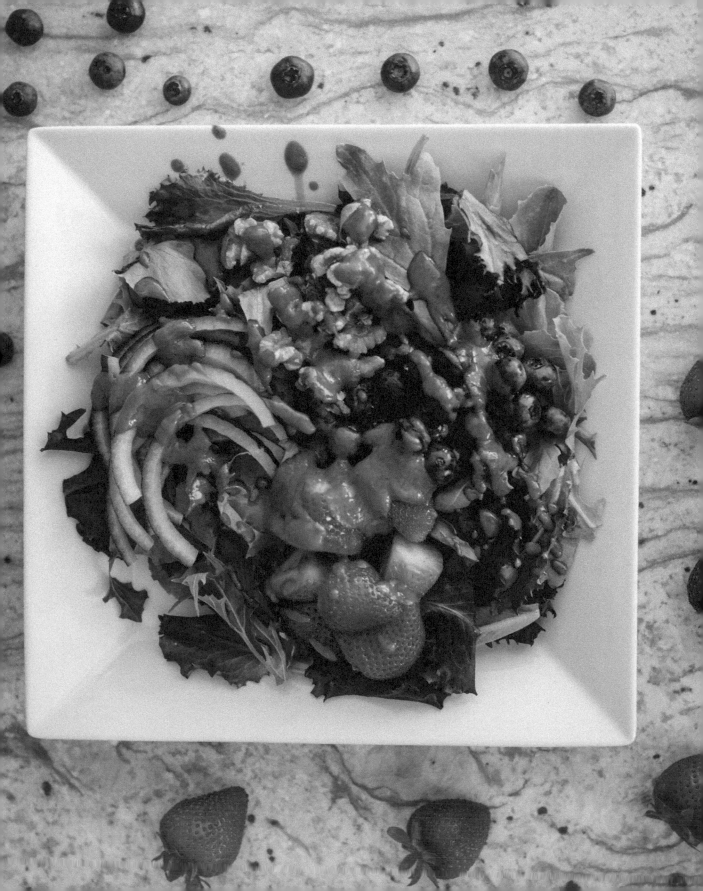

// *Opposite:* Berry Green
Salad (PAGE 97)

Sides

BAKED BEANS

YIELDS 4 SERVINGS

PREP TIME: 10 minutes
COOK TIME: 5 hours

454 g white pea beans

¼ cup ketchup
(recipe on page 47)

¼ cup blackstrap molasses

2 tbsp organic mustard

1 tsp garlic powder

1 tsp onion powder

¼ tsp pepper

Baked beans were a regular fixture on my childhood dinner table. My mother would often cook them as a main meal, but my British husband was raised pairing beans as a side with other foods. Since we met, we have greatly enjoyed eating these beauty beans with another Newfoundland favourite—fish cakes! The two go together perfectly, so be sure to try this wholesome, healthy baked-bean recipe with the Cauliflower Cod Cakes on page 72!

1   Add beans to a large pot and cover with water. Boil for 1 hour. You may need to add extra water as they cook, so make sure you check occasionally.

2   Pour boiled beans and water into roaster.

3   Preheat oven to 325°F.

4   Pour extra water in roaster until about halfway full.

5   Add the remaining ingredients and stir until well combined.

6   Bake in oven for 4 hours.

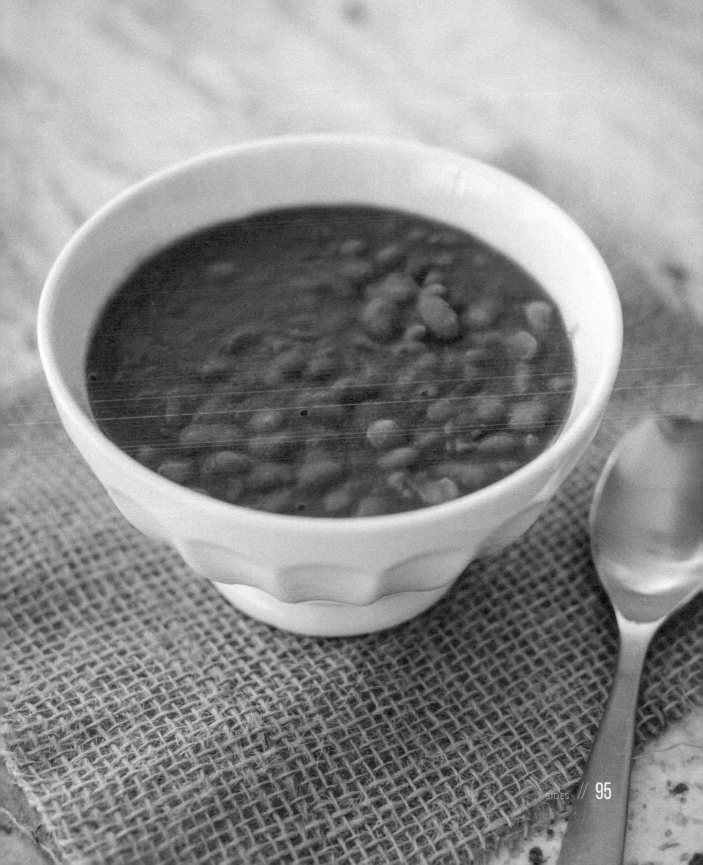

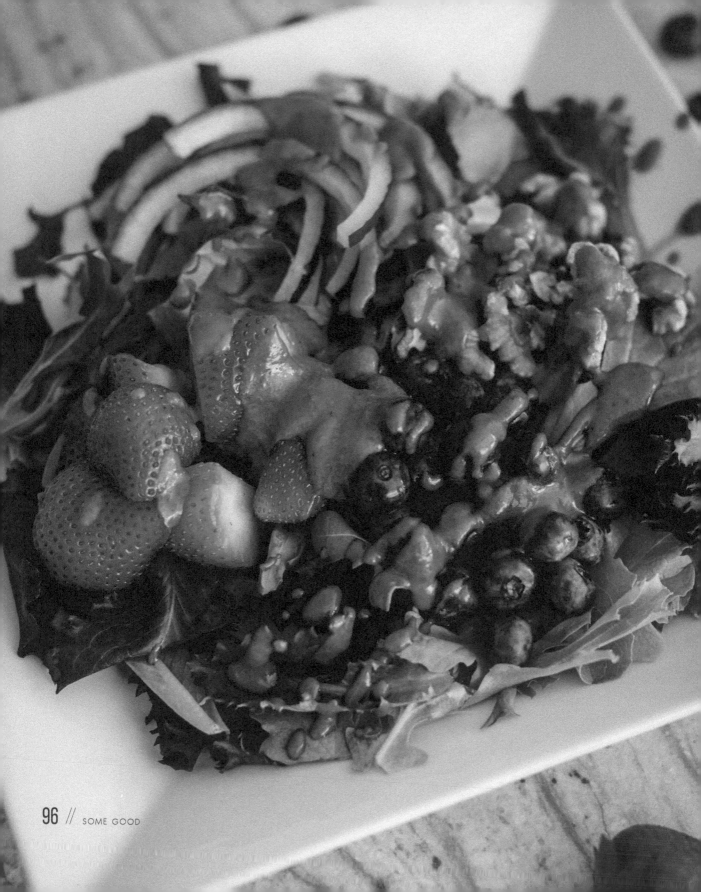

BERRY GREEN SALAD

Berries are so abundant in Newfoundland and Labrador. We truly are blessed to have so much of nature's candy growing freely everywhere we turn. Adding these sweet treats to a bed of leafy greens, along with some veggies and nuts, makes for a really great tasting salad!

1 Place mixed greens in a bowl or plate.

2 Add onion, strawberries, blueberries, and walnuts to greens and toss.

3 Serve with Partridgeberry Salad Dressing (found on page 54).

SERVES 1 AS MAIN MEAL, 2 AS A SIDE

PREP TIME: 10 minutes

4 cups loosely packed mixed greens

¼ red onion, sliced thinly

¼ cup sliced strawberries

¼ cup blueberries

¼ cup chopped walnuts

ROASTED VEGGIES

YIELDS 4 SIDE SERVINGS

PREP TIME: 15 minutes
COOK TIME: 45 minutes

- 2 sweet potatoes, largely diced
- 1 small onion, sliced
- 4 carrots, halved and largely diced
- 1 small turnip, largely diced
- ¼ large cabbage, roughly chopped
- 6 tbsp extra-virgin olive oil
- 2 tbsp thyme
- ½ tsp sea salt
- dash pepper

While it's traditional to boil your vegetables in Newfoundland, for Jiggs or Sunday Dinner, the boiling process can destroy many of the nutrients in your vegetables. Roasting these tasty Newfoundland favourites really maximizes their taste while giving them a satisfying crispy texture, plus you get to keep all those lovely nutrients.

1 Preheat oven to 375°F.

2 Place all vegetables in glass baking dish. Drizzle with oil and sprinkle herbs and spices.

3 Bake for 45 to 50 minutes or until vegetables are tender, stirring vegetables halfway through baking time.

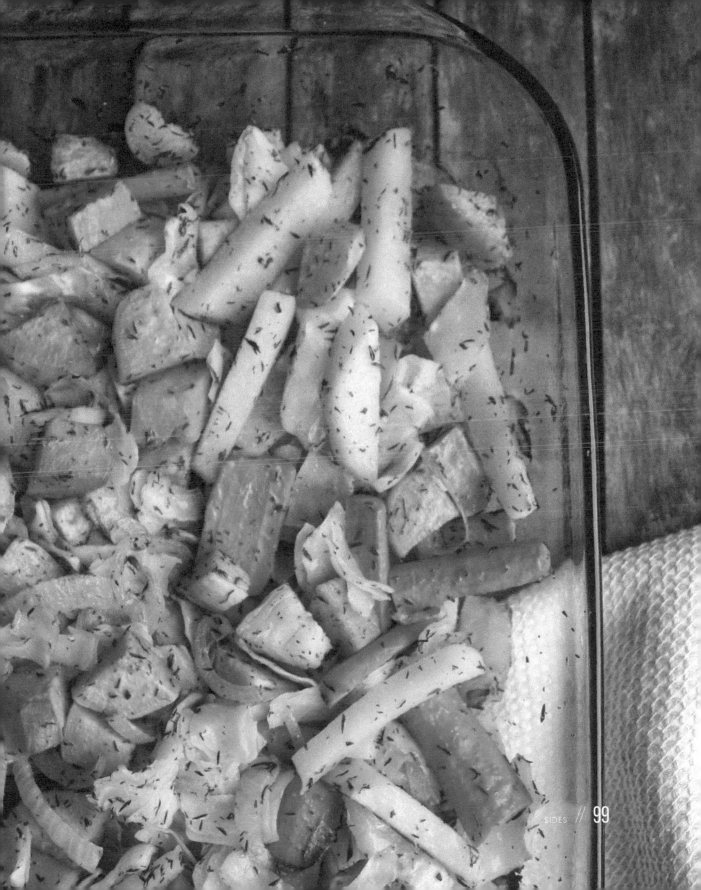

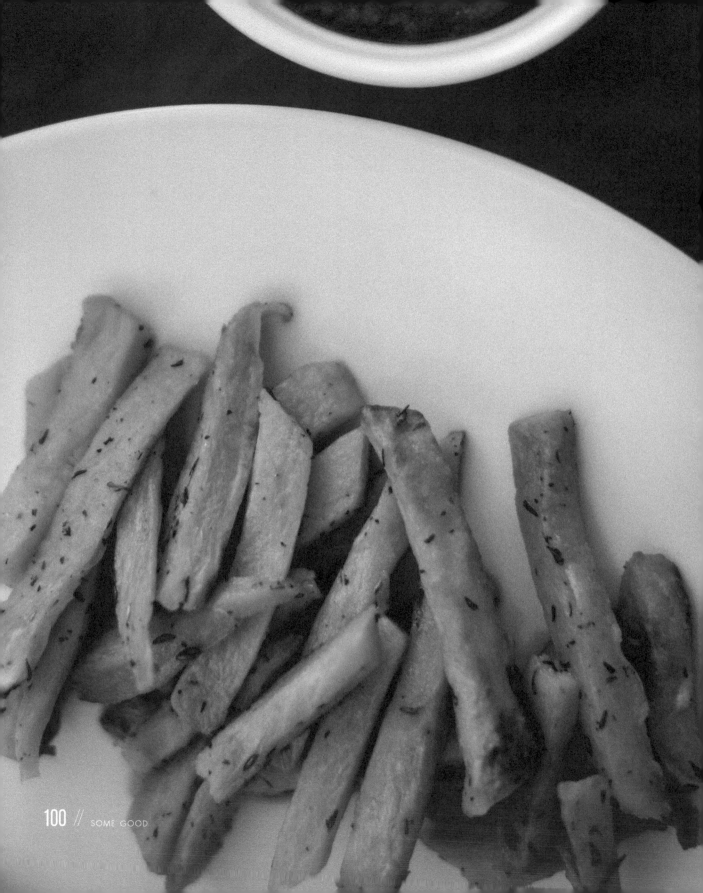

SWEET POTATO FRIES

YIELDS 2 SERVINGS

PREP TIME: 10 minutes
COOK TIME: 24 minutes

Because you can't have battered fish without fries! Sweet potatoes make for delicious, sweet fries that go great with the Battered Baked Cod you'll find on page 85. Fish and Chips—one of the most famous traditional Newfoundland dishes—completely reimagined to be cleaner, healthier, and just as delicious!

1 large sweet potato, peeled and sliced into thin sticks

2 tbsp extra-virgin olive oil

½ tsp sea salt

½ tsp thyme

¼ tsp pepper

1 Preheat oven to 375°F.

2 Place all ingredients into medium bowl and toss to cover sweet potatoes entirely.

3 Place sweet potatoes on baking sheet and bake for 20 minutes. After 20 minutes, broil fries for 4 minutes or until golden brown on top.

BEET-IFUL COLESLAW

½ **head cabbage**

2 **beets, raw**

2 **carrots**

1 **small apple, peeled and finely chopped**

1 **cup cashews, soaked for at least 6 hours or overnight**

½ **cup water**

1 **tbsp apple-cider vinegar**

2 **tbsp honey**

Beets are such a beautiful and vibrant vegetable. They are great roasted, bottled, and even raw! If you are new to raw beets, this delicious Beet-iful Coleslaw is a great way to enjoy them in their most naked form. Phenomenal flavours, and so pretty in colour!

1 Core and shred cabbage. Place in bowl.

2 Peel and shred carrots and beets. Place in bowl.

3 Add apple to vegetable mixture and set aside.

4 Place cashews and water in blender and blend to a smooth consistency. Transfer cashew cream to bowl, add vinegar and honey, and thoroughly combine.

5 Add cashew mixture to coleslaw and thoroughly combine.

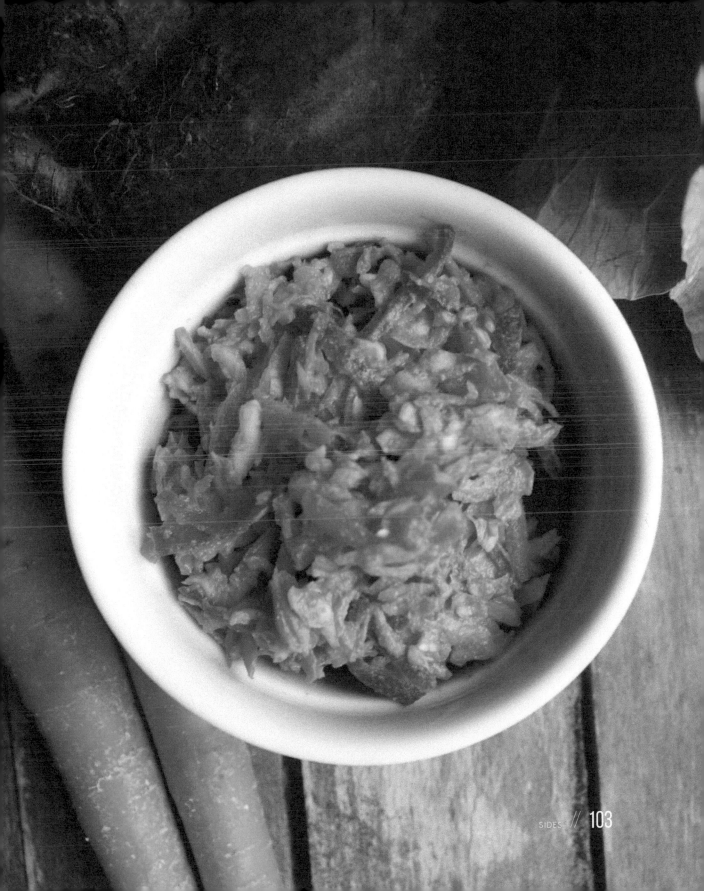

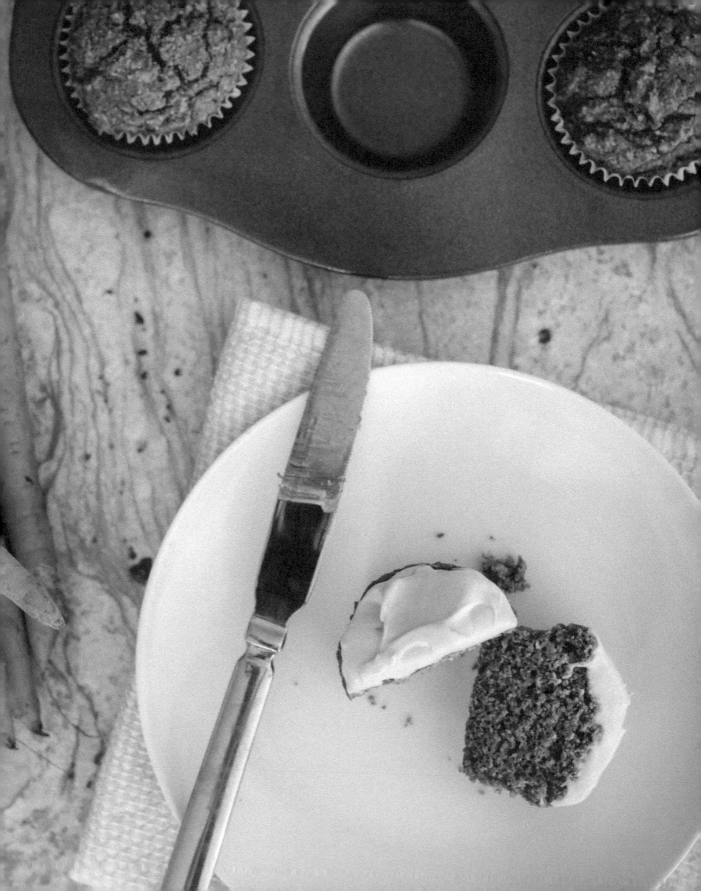

Desserts

BLUEBERRY COTTAGE PUDDING

YIELDS 9 SERVINGS

PREP TIME: 15 minutes
COOK TIME: 30 minutes

1¾ cups brown rice flour

2½ tsp baking powder

½ tsp sea salt

½ cup coconut sugar

¼ cup coconut oil, melted

1 egg

1 tsp vanilla

⅔ cup almond milk

1 cup fresh or frozen blueberries

Puddings are a favourite of mine. So dense and moist, they are a sweet, satisfying, and flavourful dessert. Adding a Newfoundland berry to the mix makes this pudding that much more delicious. While many traditional puddings are made with refined sugars and flours, this Blueberry Cottage Pudding offers a whole lot of wholefood goodness!

1   Preheat oven to 350°F and grease 8 x 8 baking dish with coconut oil.

2   Combine flour, baking powder, salt, and sugar together.

3   Add the oil, egg, vanilla, and milk. Mix until thoroughly combined.

4   Lastly, add the blueberries and thoroughly combine.

5   Pour mixture into the greased baking dish and bake for 30 minutes.

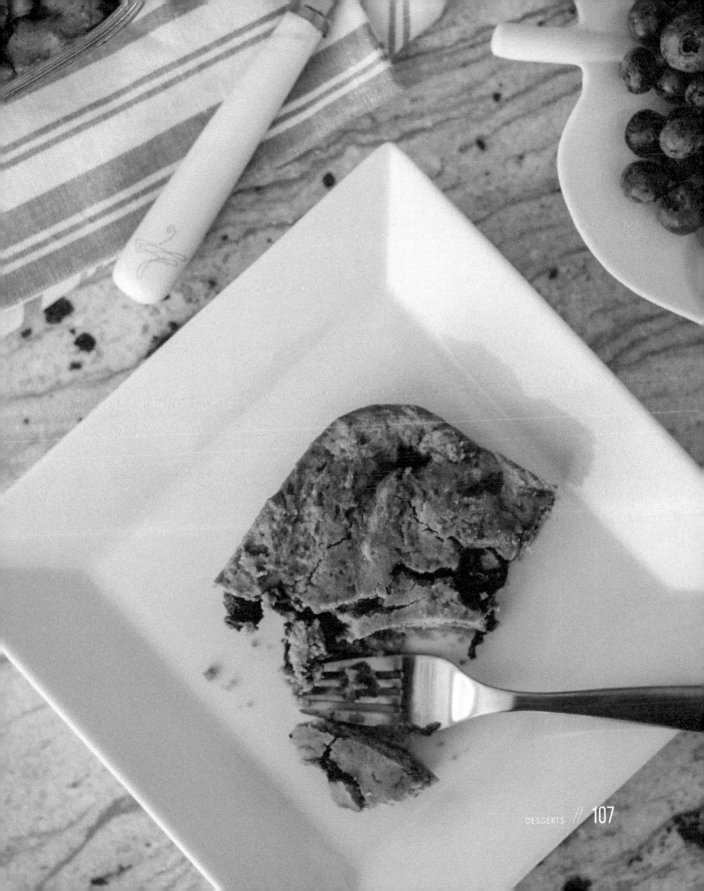

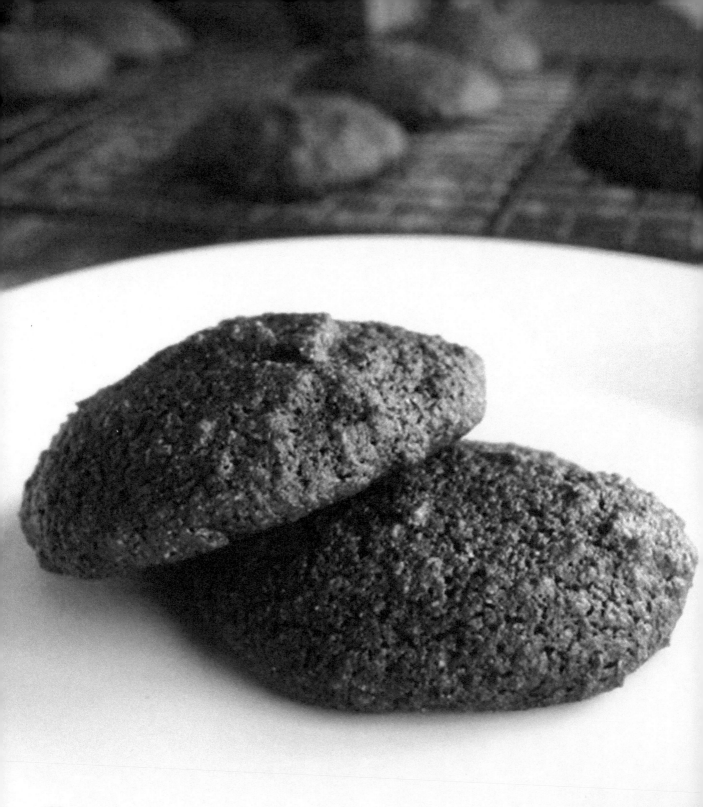

MOLASSES COOKIES

YIELDS 28 COOKIES

PREP TIME: 15 minutes
COOK TIME: 10 minutes

My grandmother made molasses cookies all the time, and they were a huge hit with my taste buds as a child. The flavour was so sweet and distinctive, and will always take me right back to her kitchen. My Molasses Cookies offer all that unique molasses goodness and spice-infused flavour, without any of the refined ingredients.

- ¾ cup buckwheat flour
- ¾ cup brown rice flour
- ½ cup almond flour
- 1 tsp cinnamon
- 1 tsp ground ginger
- 1 tsp baking powder
- ½ cup coconut sugar
- ¼ cup almond milk
- 1 egg
- ½ cup blackstrap molasses
- ¼ cup coconut oil, melted
- 2 tbsp unsweetened applesauce

1 Preheat oven to 350°F and place parchment paper on a cookie sheet.

2 Combine flours, cinnamon, ginger, and baking powder together in a bowl.

3 In another bowl, whisk together coconut sugar, almond milk, egg, blackstrap molasses, coconut oil, and applesauce.

4 Gradually add the dry mixture to the wet mixture until thoroughly combined.

5 Use a tablespoon to spoon mixture onto cookie sheet to make cookies.

6 Bake for 10 minutes.

DATE SQUARES

YIELDS 1 SQUARE
BAKING DISH

PREP TIME: 20 minutes
COOK TIME: 35 minutes

2 cups dates

1 cup water

½ cup coconut sugar

1½ cup brown rice flour

½ tsp baking soda

1 tsp baking powder

¼ tsp sea salt

1 cup coconut oil

1½ cup rolled oats

Whenever I think of date squares, I am immediately reminded of my father. Ever since I was small, he would ask Mom to make them, and he still enjoys them to this day. While it took me a while to warm to Dad's preferred dessert, these days I do appreciate the virtues of a good date square. I hope you come to love my healthier take on them, too!

1 Remove pits from dates, coarsely chop the dates, and add to saucepan with water.

2 Simmer until thick, around 5 to 10 minutes, and let cool.

3 Preheat oven to 325°F and grease an 8 x 8 glass baking dish.

4 Combine flour, baking powder, soda, and salt. Drop pieces of coconut oil into flour mixture.

5 Add coconut sugar and rolled oats, then combine.

6 Place ¾ of the oat mixture in baking dish. Then add date mixture and add the remaining oat mixture over top.

7 Bake for 35 minutes. Let cool and enjoy!

OATMEAL TARTS

YIELDS 5 TARTS

PREP TIME: 15 minutes
COOK TIME: 12 minutes

Tarts are a great way to enjoy all those delectable Newfoundland preserves. Fill them with your favourite jam and they make a fantastic snack or dessert. Try these Oatmeal Tarts with the Bakeapple Jam (on page 48). The sweet base beautifully offsets the tartness of the bakeapples. This is a fibre-filled dessert that will keep you feeling satisfied.

- ¾ cup quick rolled oats
- ¼ cup brown rice flour
- ¼ cup almond meal
- ½ tsp baking powder
- ¼ tsp sea salt
- ¼ cup honey
- 2 tbsp coconut oil, extra for greasing pan

1 Preheat oven to 350°F.

2 Combine oats, flours, baking powder, and salt together in bowl.

3 Add honey and coconut oil, and mix in well until everything is sticking together.

4 Grease cupcake pan with coconut oil and use a ¼ cup to measure out enough oat mixture into each cup.

5 Press the oat mixture up against the sides and bottom of the cupcake form to create tart.

6 Bake for 12 minutes.

CARROT MUFFINS *with* CASHEW CREAM CHEESE FROSTING

YIELDS 12 MUFFINS

PREP TIME: 15 minutes
COOK TIME: 25 minutes

dry
INGREDIENTS

¾ cup brown rice flour

¾ cup buckwheat flour

½ cup almond flour

1 tsp baking powder

1 tsp baking soda

1 tsp cinnamon

½ tsp ground ginger

½ tsp allspice

½ tsp sea salt

wet
INGREDIENTS

1 egg

½ cup maple syrup

½ cup applesauce

½ cup water

¼ cup coconut oil, melted

1 tbsp apple-cider vinegar

1 tsp vanilla extract

additional
INGREDIENTS

1½ cups shredded carrot

Carrot cake and muffins were among my favourite desserts growing up. Smothering them in a cream-cheese icing is a treasured childhood memory of mine—especially when Mom let us lick the bowl! Today, I appreciate how these lovely muffins make use of a common sweet Newfoundland root vegetable in dessert form. My Carrot Muffins are free of dairy, and refined sugar and flours, but still taste just as good as the originals.

1   Preheat oven to 350°F and line a 12-cup muffin pan with paper liners.

2   Mix all the dry ingredients together in a medium bowl and set aside.

3   Whisk all the wet ingredients together in a medium bowl.

4   Add the wet ingredients to the dry ingredients and mix until fully combined.

5   Fold in shredded carrot.

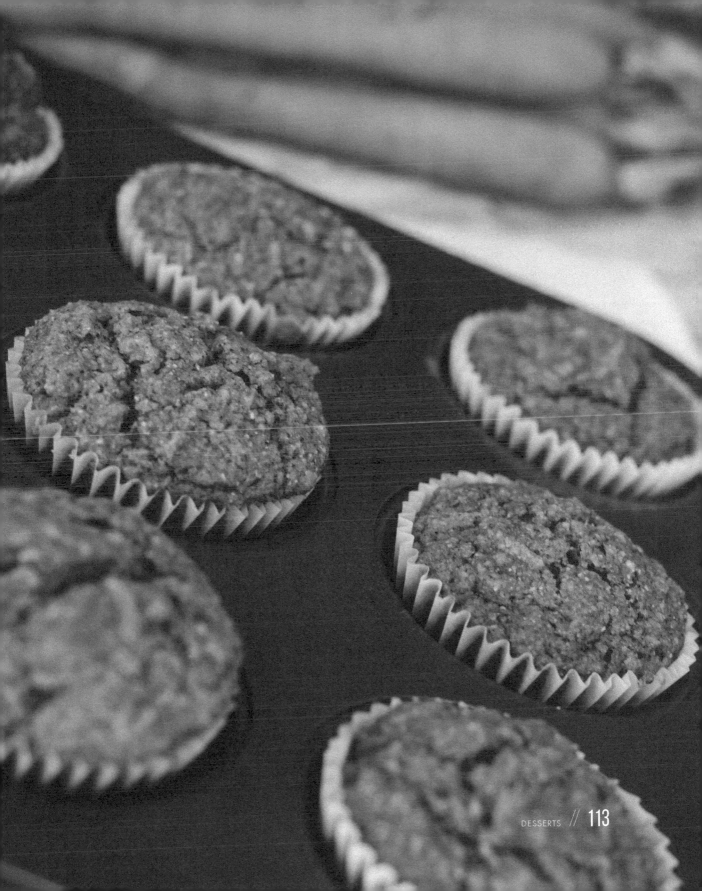

6 Use a ¼ cup measure to scoop batter out into paper liners.

7 Bake for 25 minutes, or until a toothpick inserted in the center of a muffin comes out clean.

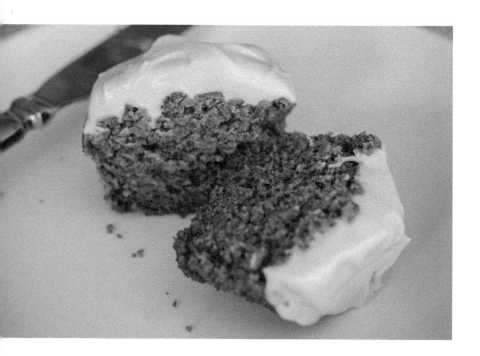

cashew cream cheese frosting

YIELDS 1 CUP

PREP TIME: 10 minutes

So creamy and delicious, this frosting makes a carrot muffin taste that much better! In fact, you can add it to pretty much any of your favourite cakes and baked goods for a tasty, creamy topping—without the dairy!

1 cup cashews, soaked for 6 hours, or overnight
3 tbsp water
2 tbsp honey
1 tsp vanilla extract

1 Add all ingredients to a blender or food processor and blend until you reach a smooth consistency.

NEWFOUNDLAND BERRY CRUMBLE

YIELDS 4 SERVINGS

PREP TIME: 15 minutes
COOK TIME: 45 minutes

I do love a good crumble. That crispy, crumbly texture works perfectly, no matter what your fruit base of choice. This particular crumble is very much Newfoundland inspired, incorporating three of Newfoundland's most famous berries: bakeapples, partridgeberries, and blueberries. Combine these beauties together and you get a memorable crumble to serve as dessert!

1　Preheat oven to 350°F.

2　Mix base ingredients together in an 8 x 8 baking dish.

3　Combine topping ingredients in a small bowl and crumble on top of berry mixture.

4　Bake for 45 minutes.

base
INGREDIENTS

1 cup bakeapples

1 cup partridgeberries

1 cup blueberries

¼ cup honey

½ tsp arrowroot flour

topping
INGREDIENTS

¾ cup rolled oats

½ cup brown rice flour

½ tsp cinnamon

¼ cup honey

2 tbsp coconut oil

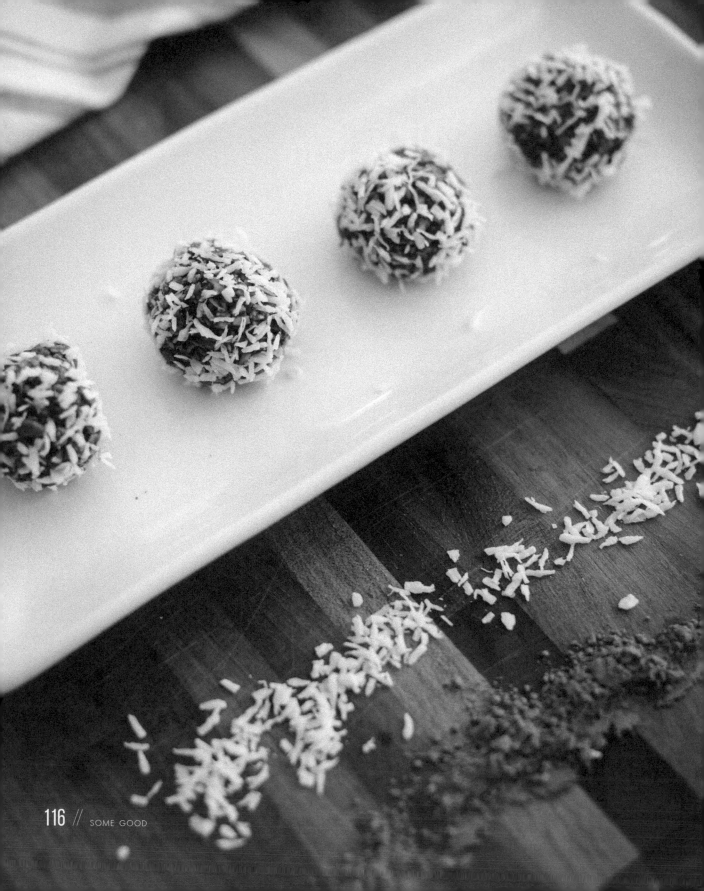

SNOWBALLS

My childhood involved two types of snowballs. The first kind was cold and stung when it hit you in the face. The second kind was much sweeter and made you smile when you stuffed it in your face! My mother made snowballs every Christmas and they are, for me, synonymous with the holiday season. Personally, I've always preferred my snowballs ice cold, straight out of the freezer. Maybe it's something to do with the name...

1 Melt coconut oil, almond milk, sugar, and cacao powder together over medium heat in a medium-sized pot.

2 Once melted and ingredients are combined, remove from burner and stir in vanilla.

3 Add ½ cup of coconut and rolled oats, and combine ingredients.

4 With a tablespoon measure, scoop out mixture and roll into small balls. Then roll balls into the remainder of coconut to coat the outside.

5 Place balls on a cookie sheet lined with parchment paper and let chill in refrigerator for 1 hour.

6 These can be stored in the refrigerator or freezer.

YIELDS 28 BALLS

PREP TIME: 15 minutes
COOK TIME: 5 minutes + 1 hour chilling time

½ cup coconut oil

½ cup almond milk

½ cup coconut sugar

3 tbsp cacao powder

1 tsp vanilla extract

½ cup coconut, plus ½ cup for rolling

2½ cups rolled oats

HEALTHY HERMITS

YIELDS 12 COOKIES

PREP TIME: 10 minutes
COOK TIME: 15 minutes

½ cup brown rice flour

¼ cup buckwheat flour

1 cup rolled oats

½ tsp baking soda

½ tsp sea salt

½ tsp nutmeg

½ tsp cinnamon

½ tsp Dandy Blend

½ cup walnuts, chopped

½ cup unsweetened
   dried cranberries,
   chopped

½ cup coconut oil, melted

½ cup coconut sugar

1 egg

¼ cup water

My mother would bake these cake-like cookies every time my father was going in the woods to hunt or fish—a tradition they maintain to this day! The variety of ingredients in these cookies creates a really interesting taste experience, and the texture is very satisfying. This is a delicious and fibre-filled treat!

1   Preheat oven to 350°F and line a large baking sheet with parchment paper.

2   Combine flours, oats, baking soda, salt, nutmeg, cinnamon, Dandy Blend, walnuts, and cranberries in a medium bowl, and set aside.

3   Combine oil, coconut sugar, egg, and water together in a separate bowl.

4   Add the wet ingredients to the dry ingredients and thoroughly combine.

5   Use a heaping tablespoon to make cookies and place on cookie sheet.

6   Bake for 15 minutes.

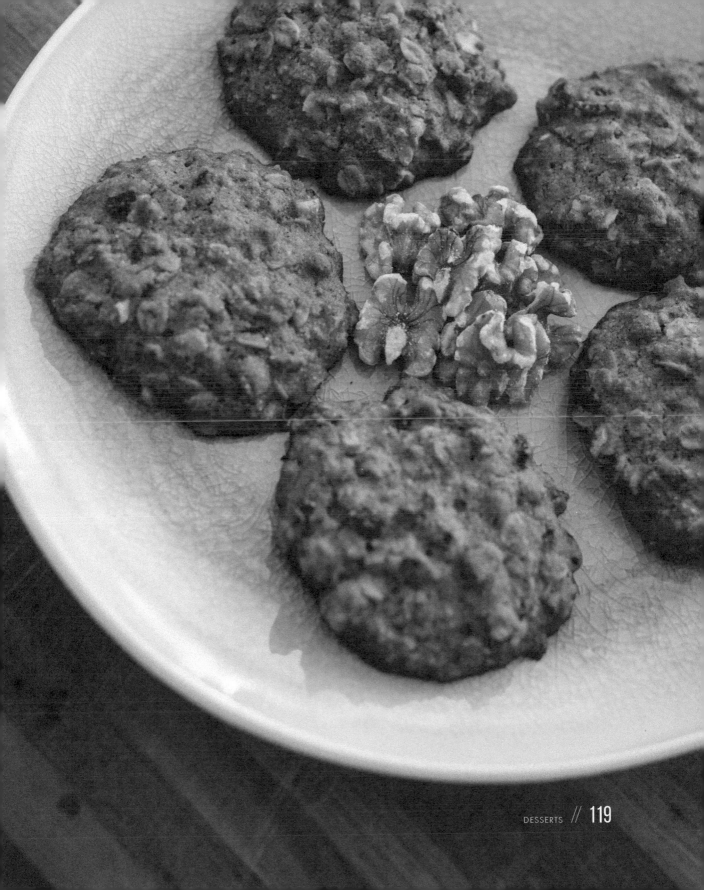

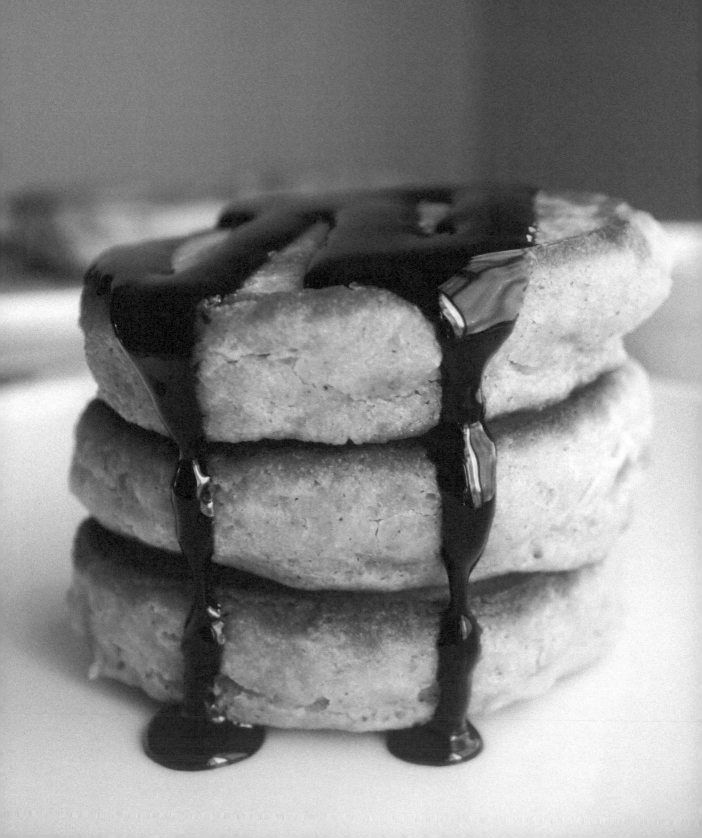

Opposite: Toutons (page 125)

Breads

NO-KNEAD BREAD

PREP TIME: 4 hours 15 minutes
COOK TIME: 45 minutes

1 cup brown rice flour

1 cup sorghum flour

1 cup oat flour

½ cup arrowroot flour

1 tsp sea salt

1 tbsp coconut sugar

1½ tsp active-dry yeast

2 eggs

1–1½ cups lukewarm water

½ tbsp sesame seeds
   (optional)

**Coconut oil for
   greasing the loaf pan**

As if homemade bread without the need to knead wasn't great news enough, this bread is also gluten-free, elevating it to 'must make' status! When picking out yeast for this wondrous bread recipe, make sure you get one that is gluten and additive free. One common additive in active dry yeast is sorbitan monostearate—a nasty emulsifier also known as synthetic wax. Stay away from such additives and look for an active dry yeast with just 'yeast' in the ingredients. Serve a slice of toasted No-Knead Bread covered in Homemade Bakeapple Jam (page 48), or try it with the Poached Egg and Roasted Veggies found on page 60.

1 Place all flours, sea salt, coconut sugar, and active dry yeast in a medium bowl and whisk until thoroughly combined. Set aside.

2 Whisk eggs in a separate small bowl and pour eggs over flour mixture.

3 Use a bit of elbow grease to mix flour and eggs.

4 Gradually pour in water a little bit at a time. Combine ingredients together with hands until you reach a thick and sticky dough-like texture.

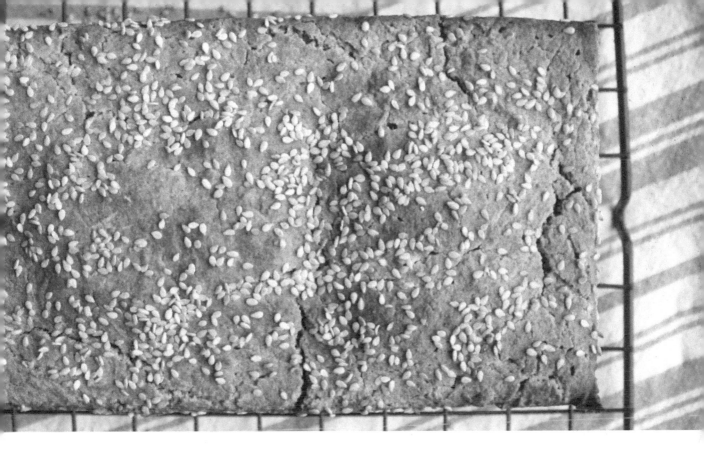

5   When ingredients are thoroughly combined, pour dough into a glass bowl and cover with a clean dish towel.

6   Place bowl in a warm place in your home. Let dough rise for 2 hours.

7   **AFTER 2 HOURS OF RISING IN THE BOWL:** Transfer dough to a greased 9" x 5" loaf pan. Cover with clean dish towel and let rise again for 1 hour and 30 minutes to 2 hours. (Rising time may vary depending on where you live and how warm it is in your home.)

8   Preheat oven to 450°F.

9   With a pastry brush, gently brush lukewarm water over loaf and sprinkle with sesame seeds for decoration. This is optional.

10 Once oven has reached temperature, bake for 45 minutes.

11 Once baked, remove from oven and place on cooling rack. After 10 minutes, your bread should start to remove itself from the sides of the loaf pan. Remove bread loaf from loaf pan and let cool on cooling rack for another hour before slicing.

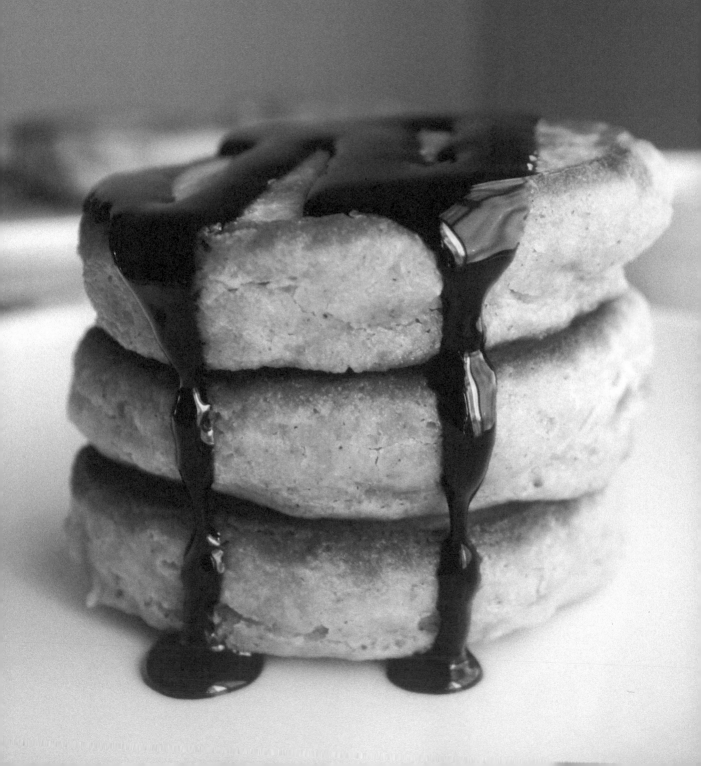

TOUTONS

Nothing says 'Newfoundland and Labrador' like a good ol' touton, or fried bread dough. Instead of making a loaf of the No-Knead Bread, use the mixture to fry yourself up some delicious, gluten-free toutons. They make a great accompaniment to breakfast and are always a treat with a drizzle of molasses or maple syrup.

1 Heat coconut oil in pan on medium heat.

2 Use a ¼ cup measure to scoop out bread dough and place in heated pan.

3 Fry bread for about 2-3 minutes or until golden brown. Flip touton and fry other side for 2-3 minutes or until golden brown.

4 Drizzle with blackstrap molasses or maple syrup. Enjoy!

YIELDS 9 SERVINGS

PREP TIME: 5 minutes
COOK TIME: 8 minutes

No-Knead Bread Dough
   (recipe on page 122), **risen for 4 hours in glass bowl**

2 tbsp coconut oil

PEA SUPER SOUP DUMPLINGS

YIELDS 6 SERVINGS

PREP TIME: 5 minutes
COOK TIME: 15 minutes

- ½ cup plus 2 tbsp brown rice flour
- ½ cup plus 2 tbsp sorghum flour
- ½ cup arrowroot flour
- 1 tsp sea salt
- 2 tsp baking powder
- 1 cup cold water

Pea soup is not pea soup without the dumplings! They're the icing on the cake for pea soup! A quick and easy dumpling that is gluten-free to help you stay away from those refined flours, these dumplings are best served bobbing around in the Pea Super Soup on page 75.

1 When Pea Super Soup has 20 minutes of cook time left, whisk flours, sea salt and baking powder in a bowl.

2 Add cold water and stir until thoroughly combined. Using a spoon, drop the dumpling mixture into the Pea Super Soup.

3 Place cover over soup and dumplings and let simmer for 15 minutes. It is important to keep the cover on the pot during this cooking time.

4 Once cooked, you can remove dumplings from the pot and place on a plate to serve with Pea Super Soup. Enjoy!

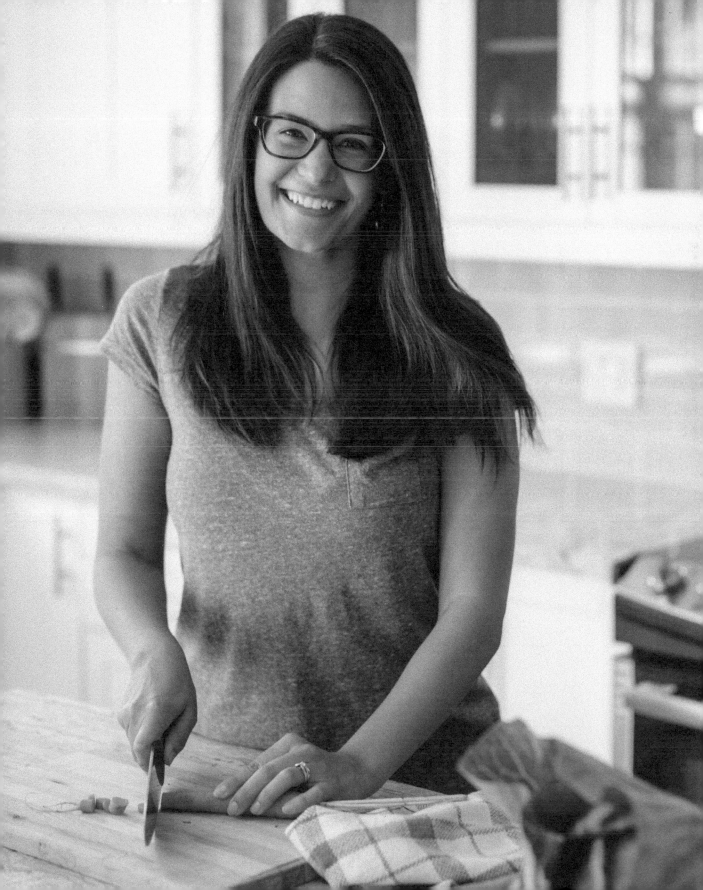

MEASUREMENT TABLES
approximated

DRY MEASURES

1 oz	=	28 g
2 oz	=	57 g
3 oz	=	85 g
4 oz	=	113 g
6 oz	=	170 g
8 oz	=	227 g
12 oz	=	340 g
16 oz	=	454 g
32 oz	=	907 g

LIQUID MEASUREMENTS

3 tsp	1 tbsp	½ fl oz	15 ml
2 tbsp	⅛ cup	1 fl oz	30 ml
4 tbsp	¼ cup	2 fl oz	60 ml
8 tbsp	½ cup	4 fl oz	115 ml
12 tbsp	¾ cup	6 fl oz	150 ml
16 tbsp	1 cup	8 fl oz	237 ml
32 tbsp	2 cups	16 fl oz	474 ml

ENDNOTES

1   Jenny Higgins, "20th-Century Fisheries and Settlement Patterns," Heritage
    Newfoundland and Labrador, accessed March 25, 2017,
    http://www.heritage.nf.ca/articles/economy/20th-century-fishery.php.

2   Keith Collier, "Malnutrition in Newfoundland and Labrador," Heritage
    Newfoundland and Labrador, accessed March 25, 2017,
    http://www.heritage.nf.ca/articles/society/malnutrition.php.

3   Elson M. Haas and Buck Levin, *Staying Healthy with Nutrition: The Complete Guide
    to Diet and Nutritional Medicine* (Berkeley: Celestial Arts, 2006), 143.

4   Keith Collier, "Malnutrition in Newfoundland and Labrador," Heritage
    Newfoundland and Labrador, accessed March 25, 2017,
    http://www.heritage.nf.ca/articles/society/malnutrition.php; Elson M. Haas and Buck
    Levin, *Staying Healthy with Nutrition: The Complete Guide to Diet and Nutritional
    Medicine* (Berkeley: Celestial Arts, 2006), 100.

5   Keith Collier, "Malnutrition in Newfoundland and Labrador," Heritage
    Newfoundland and Labrador, accessed March 25, 2017,
    http://www.heritage.nf.ca/articles/society/malnutrition.php.

6   Michael Moss, *Salt, Sugar, Fat: How the Food Giants Hooked Us* (London: WH
    Allen, 2014), 9-12, 157, 174, 255.

7   Cod," The World's Healthiest Foods, accessed March 25, 2017,
    http://www.whfoods.com/genpage.php?tname=foodspice&dbid=133.

8   Disappearance of the Beothuk," Heritage Newfoundland and Labrador,
    accessed November 29, 2017, http://www.heritage.nf.ca/articles/aboriginal/
    beothuk-disappearance.php.

9   "Introduction of Moose to the Island of Newfoundland," Provincial Heritage
    Commemorations Program, accessed November 29, 2017,
    http://commemorations.ca/introduction-of-moose-to-the-island-of-newfoundland/.

10 Natalie Stein, "Moose Meat Nutritional Value," LIVESTRONG.COM, October 03, 2017, accessed November 29, 2017, https://www.livestrong.com/article/466820-moose-meat-nutritional-value/.

11 Krista Scott-Dixon and Brian St. Pierre, "Sweet vs. Regular Potatoes: Which Potatoes Are REALLY Healthier?" Precision Nutrition, January 24, 2017, accessed June 07, 2017, http://www.precisionnutrition.com/regular-vs-sweet-potatoes.

12 V. Lobo, A. Patil, A. Phatak, and N. Chandra, "Free Radicals, Antioxidants and Functional Foods: Impact on Human Health," Pharmacognosy Reviews, 2010, accessed November 29, 2017, https://www.ncbi.nlm.nih.gov/pmc/articles/PMC3249911/.

13 Phyllis A. Balch, *Prescription for Dietary Wellness* (New York: Penguin, 2003) 58-70.

14 "Winter & Summer Savory Herb: Health Benefits, Facts, Nutrition & Medicinal Uses," Home Remedies For You, accessed November 29, 2017, http://www.home-remedies-for-you.com/herbs/savory.html.

15 Government of Canada, Office of the Auditor General of Canada, "Hormones Used in Livestock Production," Government of Canada, Office of the Auditor General of Canada, accessed November 27, 2017, http://www.oag-bvg.gc.ca/internet/English/pet_203_e_28939.html.

16 Mike Ewall, "Bovine Growth Hormone: Milk Does Nobody Good...," Bovine Growth Hormone: Milk Does Nobody Good..., accessed March 25, 2017, https://www.ejnet.org/bgh/nogood.html.

17 "How Milk Gets from the Cow to the Store - Milk - ProCon.org," Is Drinking Milk Healthy for Humans? accessed April 25, 2017, https://milk.procon.org/view.resource.php?resourceID=000658.

18 Carolee Bateson-Koch, *Allergies, Disease in Disguise: How to Heal Your Allergic Condition Permanently and Naturally* (Sydney, N.S.W.: RHYW, 2010), 157-158.

19 Ibid.

20 "What Is Gluten?" Celiac Disease Foundation, accessed March 25, 2017, https://celiac.org/live-gluten-free/glutenfreediet/what-is-gluten/.

21 Ibid.

22 Justin Hollon, Elaine Leonard Puppa, Bruce Greenwald, Eric Goldberg, Anthony Guerrerio, and Alessio Fasano. "Effect of Gliadin on Permeability of Intestinal Biopsy Explants from Celiac Disease Patients and Patients with Non-Celiac Gluten Sensitivity," Nutrients, March 2015, accessed November 29, 2017, https://www.ncbi.nlm.nih.gov/pmc/articles/PMC4377866/.

23 M. Hadjivassiliou, D. G. Rao, R. A. Grinewald, D. P. Aeschlimann, P. G. Sarrigiannis, N. Hoggard, P. Aeschlimann, P. D. Mooney, and D. S. Sanders, "Neurological Dysfunction in Coeliac Disease and Non-Coeliac Gluten Sensitivity," The American Journal of Gastroenterology, April 2016, accessed March 25, 2017, https://www.ncbi.nlm.nih.gov/pubmed/26832652; Elena F. Verdu, David Armstrong, and Joseph A. Murray, "Between Celiac Disease and Irritable Bowel Syndrome: The 'No Man's Land' of Gluten Sensitivity," The American Journal of Gastroenterology, June 2009, accessed November 29, 2017, https://www.ncbi.nlm.nih.gov/pmc/articles/PMC3480312/; "Gluten Sensitivity as a Neurological Illness − Hadjivassiliou," Scribd, accessed November 29, 2017, https://www.scribd.com/document/363068140/Gluten-Sensitivity-as-a-Nurological-Illness-Hadjivassiliou; Jessica R. Biesiekierski and Julie Iven, "Non-coeliac Gluten Sensitivity: Piecing the Puzzle Together," United European Gastroenterology Journal, April 2015, accessed November 29, 2017, https://www.ncbi.nlm.nih.gov/pmc/articles/PMC4406911/.

24 Nicole M. Avena, Pedro Rada, and Bartley G. Hoebel, "Evidence for Sugar Addiction: Behavioral and Neurochemical Effects of Intermittent, Excessive Sugar Intake," Neuroscience and Biobehavioral Reviews, 2008, accessed November 29, 2017, https://www.ncbi.nlm.nih.gov/pmc/articles/PMC2235907/.

25 James J. DiNicolantonio and Amy Berger, "Added Sugars Drive Nutrient and Energy Deficit in Obesity: A New Paradigm," Open Heart, 2016, accessed April 25, 2018, https://www.ncbi.nlm.nih.gov/pmc/articles/PMC4975866/.

26 Ibid.

27 "About Glycemic Index," The University of Sydney, accessed November 29, 2017, http://www.glycemicindex.com/about.php.

28 Elson M. Haas and Buck Levin, Staying Healthy with Nutrition: The Complete Guide to Diet and Nutritional Medicine (Berkeley: Celestial Arts, 2006), 112.

29 V. Lobo, A. Patil, A. Phatak, and N. Chandra, "Free Radicals, Antioxidants and Functional Foods: Impact on Human Health," Pharmacognosy Reviews, 2010, accessed November 29, 2017, https://www.ncbi.nlm.nih.gov/pmc/articles/PMC3249911/; Lois Baker, "Study Shows Glucose Consumption Increases Production of Destructive Free Radicals, Lowers Level of Key Antioxidant," Study Shows Glucose Consumption Increases Production of Destructive Free Radicals, Lowers Level of Key Antioxidant - University at Buffalo, August 16, 2000, accessed March 25, 2017, http://www.buffalo.edu/news/releases/2000/08/4839.html.

30 "About Glycemic Index," The University of Sydney, accessed November 29, 2017, http://www.glycemicindex.com/about.php.

REFERENCES

"About Glycemic Index." The University of Sydney. Accessed November 29, 2017. http://www.glycemicindex.com/about.php.

"Almonds." The World's Healthiest Foods. Accessed November 29, 2017. http://www.whfoods.com/genpage.php?tname=foodspice&dbid=20.

Avena, Nicole M., Pedro Rada, and Bartley G. Hoebel. "Evidence for Sugar Addiction: Behavioral and Neurochemical Effects of Intermittent, Excessive Sugar Intake." Neuroscience and Biobehavioral Reviews. 2008. Accessed November 29, 2017. https://www.ncbi.nlm.nih.gov/pmc/articles/PMC2235907/.

Axe, Josh. "Raw Honey: Get More Energy (Just Like Ancient Greek Athletes Did!)." Dr. Axe. April 13, 2018. Accessed March 25, 2017. https://draxe.com/the-many-health-benefits-of-raw-honey/.

Baker, Lois. "Study Shows Glucose Consumption Increases Production of Destructive Free Radicals, Lowers Level of Key Antioxidant." University at Buffalo News Center. August 16, 2000. Accessed March 25, 2017. http://www.buffalo.edu/news/releases/2000/08/4839.html.

Balch, Phyllis A. *Prescription for Nutritional Healing: The A-to-Z Guide to Supplements.* New York: Avery, 2010.

Bateson-Koch, Carolee. *Allergies, Disease in Disguise: How to Heal Your Allergic Condition Permanently and Naturally.* Sydney: RHYW, 2010.

Biesiekierski, Jessica R., and Julie Iven. "Non-coeliac Gluten Sensitivity: Piecing the Puzzle Together." United European Gastroenterology Journal. April 2015. Accessed November 29, 2017. https://www.ncbi.nlm.nih.gov/pmc/articles/PMC4406911/.

"Brown Rice." The World's Healthiest Foods. Accessed November 29, 2017. http://www.whfoods.com/genpage.php?tname=foodspice&dbid=128.

"Buckwheat." The World's Healthiest Foods. Accessed November 29, 2017.
http://www.whfoods.com/genpage.php?tname=foodspice&dbid=11.

"Cane Sugar Refining." The Canadian Sugar Institute. Accessed March 25, 2017.
http://www.sugar.ca/Nutrition-Information-Service/Educators-Students/
Purification-of-Sugar/Cane-Sugar-Refining.aspx.

Carr, Anitra, and Silvia Maggini. "Vitamin C and Immune Function." MDPI.
November 03, 2017. Accessed November 29, 2017.
http://www.mdpi.com/2072-6643/9/11/1211/htm.

"Casein: The Disturbing Connection Between This Dairy Protein and Your Health."
One Green Planet. Accessed March 25, 2017.
http://www.onegreenplanet.org/natural-health/casein-dairy-protein-and-
your-health/.

Catassi, Carlo. "Gluten Sensitivity." Annals of Nutrition and Metabolism. November
26, 2015. Accessed November 29, 2017. https://www.karger.com/Article/
FullText/440990.

Chrysohoou, Christina, Demosthenes B. Panagiotakos, Christos Pitsavos, John
Skoumas, Xenophon Krinos, Yannis Chlopsios, Vassilios Nikolaou, and
Christodoulos Stefanadis. "Long-term Fish Consumption Is Associated with
Protection against Arrhythmia in Healthy Persons in a Mediterranean
Region-the ATTICA Study." OUP Academic. May 01, 2007. Accessed
March 25, 2017. https://academic.oup.com/ajcn/article/85/5/1385/4633154.

"Cod," The World's Healthiest Foods. Accessed March 25, 2017.
http://www.whfoods.com/genpage.php?tname=foodspice&dbid=133.

Coleman, Erin. "Myth or Fact: Brown Sugar Is Better Than White Sugar." Fit Day.
Accessed March 25, 2017. https://www.fitday.com/fitness-articles/nutrition/
healthy-eating/myth-or-fact-brown-sugar-is-better-than-white-sugar.html.

Collier, Keith. "Malnutrition in Newfoundland and Labrador." Heritage
Newfoundland and Labrador. Accessed March 25, 2017.
http://www.heritage.nf.ca/articles/society/malnutrition.php.

Davis, William. Wheat Belly: Lose the Wheat, Lose the Weight and Find Your Path
Back to Health. London: Harper Thorsons, 2015.

DiNicolantonio, James J., and Amy Berger. "Added Sugars Drive Nutrient and
Energy Deficit in Obesity: A New Paradigm." Open Heart. 2016. Accessed
November 29, 2017. https://www.ncbi.nlm.nih.gov/pmc/articles/PMC4975866/.

"Disappearance of the Beothuk." Heritage Newfoundland and Labrador.
Accessed November 29, 2017.
http://www.heritage.nf.ca/articles/aboriginal/beothuk-disappearance.php.

Ewall, Mike. "Bovine Growth Hormone: Milk Does Nobody Good." Bovine Growth Hormone: Milk Does Nobody Good. Accessed March 25, 2017. https://www.ejnet.org/bgh/nogood.html.

Government of Canada, Health Canada, and Public Affairs. "Health Canada." Veterinary Drugs Directorate—Health Canada. August 11, 2009. Accessed November 27, 2017. http://www.hc-sc.gc.ca/contact/dhp-mps/hpfb-dgpsa/vdd-dmv-eng.php.

Government of Canada, Office of the Auditor General of Canada. "Hormones Used in Livestock Production." Government of Canada, Office of the Auditor General of Canada. Accessed November 27, 2017. http://www.oag-bvg.gc.ca/internet/English/pet_203_o_28939.html.

Haas, Elson M., and Buck Levin. *Staying Healthy with Nutrition: The Complete Guide to Diet and Nutritional Medicine.* Berkeley: Celestial Arts, 2006.

Hadjivassiliou, M., R.A. Grünewald, and G.A.B. Davies-Jones. "Gluten Sensitivity as a Nurological Illness." SCRIBD. Accessed November 29, 2017. https://www.scribd.com/document/363068140/Gluten-Sensitivity-as-a-Nurological-Illness-Hadjivassiliou.

Hadjivassiliou, Marios, Dasappaiah G. Rao, Richard A. Grinewald, Daniel P. Aeschlimann, Ptolemaios G. Sarrigiannis, Nigel Hoggard, Pascale Aeschlimann, Peter D. Mooney, and David S. Sanders. "Neurological Dysfunction in Coeliac Disease and Non-Coeliac Gluten Sensitivity." Nature News. February 02, 2016. Accessed March 25, 2017. https://www.nature.com/articles/ajg201543.

Health Canada. "Veterinary Drugs." Canada.ca. January 8, 2013. Accessed November 27, 2017. https://www.canada.ca/en/health-canada/services/drugs-health-products/veterinary-drugs.html.

Higgins, Jenny. "20th-Century Fisheries and Settlement Patterns." Heritage Newfoundland and Labrador. Accessed March 25, 2017. http://www.heritage.nf.ca/articles/economy/20th-century-fishery.php.

Hollon, Justin, Elaine Leonard Puppa, Bruce Greenwald, Eric Goldberg, Anthony Guerrerio, and Alessio Fasano. "Effect of Gliadin on Permeability of Intestinal Biopsy Explants from Celiac Disease Patients and Patients with Non-Celiac Gluten Sensitivity." Nutrients. March 2015. Accessed November 29, 2017. https://www.ncbi.nlm.nih.gov/pmc/articles/PMC4377866/.

"How Milk Gets from the Cow to the Store." ProCon.org. Accessed March 25, 2017. https://milk.procon.org/view.resource.php?resourceID=000658.

"LCT Gene—Genetics Home Reference." U.S. National Library of Medicine. Accessed March 25, 2017. https://ghr.nlm.nih.gov/gene/LCT.

Lenoir, Magalie, Fuschia Serre, Lauriane Cantin, and Serge H. Ahmed. "Intense Sweetness Surpasses Cocaine Reward." PLOS ONE. Accessed March 25, 2017. http://journals.plos.org/plosone/article?id=10.1371/journal.pone.0000698.

Lobo, V., A. Patil, A. Phatak, and N. Chandra. "Free Radicals, Antioxidants and Functional Foods: Impact on Human Health." Pharmacognosy Reviews. 2010. Accessed November 29, 2017. https://www.ncbi.nlm.nih.gov/pmc/articles/PMC3249911/.

"Maple Syrup Nutrition." Pure Canadian Maple Syrup. Accessed March 25, 2017. https://www.puremaplefromcanada.com/benefits-of-maple-syrup/maple-syrup-nutrition/.

Marshall, Ingeborg. "Hunting Tools and Techniques: Food Preparation and Storage." Heritage Newfoundland and Labrador. Accessed March 25, 2017. http://www.heritage.nf.ca/articles/aboriginal/beothuk-hunting.php.

Mocchegiani, Eugenio, Javier Romeo, Marco Malavolta, Laura Costarelli, Robertina Giacconi, Ligia-Esperanza Diaz, and Ascension Marcos. "Zinc: Dietary Intake and Impact of Supplementation on Immune Function in Elderly." Age. June 2013. Accessed June 08, 2017. https://www.ncbi.nlm.nih.gov/pmc/articles/PMC3636409/.

Moss, Michael. *Salt, Sugar, Fat: How the Food Giants Hooked Us*. London: WH Allen, 2014.

Murray, Michael T. *Diabetes and Hypoglycemia: Your Natural Guide to Healing with Diet, Vitamins, Minerals, Herbs, Exercise, and Other Natural Methods.* Rocklin, CA: Prima Pub, 1994.

"Oats." The World's Healthiest Foods. Accessed November 27, 2017. http://www.whfoods.com/genpage.php?tname=foodspice&dbid=54.

Pogue, John M. "Salt Sugar Fat: How the Food Giants Hooked Us." Baylor University Medical Center Proceedings. July 2014. Accessed November 29, 2017. https://www.ncbi.nlm.nih.gov/pmc/articles/PMC4059590/.

Rhodes, Lesley E., Hassan Shahbakhti, Richard M. Azurdia, Ralf M.W. Moison, Marie-Jose S.T. Steenwinkel, Marie I. Homburg, Michael P. Dean, F. McArdle, Gerard M.J. Beijersbergen Van Henegouwen, and Bernd Epe Arie A. Vink. "Effect of Eicosapentaenoic Acid, an Omega-3 Polyunsaturated Fatty Acid, on UVR-related Cancer Risk in Humans. An Assessment of Early Genotoxic Markers." OUP Academic. May 01, 2003. Accessed March 25, 2017. https://academic.oup.com/carcin/article/24/5/919/2390522.

Rylander, Charlotta, Torkjel M. Sandanger, Dagrun Engeset, and Eiliv Lund. "Consumption of Lean Fish Reduces the Risk of Type 2 Diabetes Mellitus: A Prospective Population Based Cohort Study of Norwegian Women." PLOS ONE. Accessed March 25, 2017. http://journals.plos.org/plosone/article?id=10.1371/journal.pone.0089845.

"Savory." Home Remedies for You. Accessed November 29, 2017. http://www.home-remedies-for-you.com/herbs/savory.html.

Scott-Dixon, Krista, and Brian St. Pierre. "Sweet vs. Regular Potatoes. Which Potatoes Are Really Healthier?" Precision Nutrition. January 24, 2017. Accessed June 07, 2017. http://www.precisionnutrition.com/regular-vs-sweet-potatoes.

"Simple Healthy Living." LIVESTRONG.COM. Accessed June 07, 2017. http://www.livestrong.com/article/466820-moose-meat-nutritional-value/.

Tinggi, Ujang. "Selenium: Its Role as Antioxidant in Human Health." Environmental Health and Preventive Medicine. March 2008. Accessed March 25, 2017. https://www.ncbi.nlm.nih.gov/pmc/articles/PMC2698273/.

University of Maryland Medical Center. "Omega-3 Fatty Acids." Genetherapy. Accessed March 25, 2017. https://www.genetherapy.me/inflammation/omega-3-fatty-acids-university-of-maryland-medical-center.php.

Vasey, Christopher. *The Acid-alkaline Diet for Optimum Health: Restore Your Health by Creating PH Balance in Your Diet.* Rochester, VT: Healing Arts Press, 2006.

Verdu, Elena F., David Armstrong, and Joseph A. Murray. "Between Celiac Disease and Irritable Bowel Syndrome: The 'No Man's Land' of Gluten Sensitivity." The American Journal of Gastroenterology. June 2009. Accessed November 29, 2017. https://www.ncbi.nlm.nih.gov/pmc/articles/PMC3480312/.

Wells, Katie. "The Benefits of Soaking Nuts and Seeds." Wellness Mama. Accessed July 27, 2016. https://wellnessmama.com/59139/soaking-nuts-seeds/.

"What Is Celiac Disease?" Celiac Disease Foundation. Accessed March 25, 2017. https://celiac.org/celiac-disease/understanding-celiac-disease-2/what-is-celiac-disease/.

"What Is Gluten?" Celiac Disease Foundation. Accessed March 25, 2017. https://celiac.org/live-gluten-free/glutenfreediet/what-is-gluten/.

"Why Synthetic Vitamins Should Be Avoided Whenever Possible." Natural Society. May 15, 2015. Accessed March 25, 2017. http://naturalsociety.com/why-synthetic-vitamins-should-be-avoided/.

RECIPE INDEX

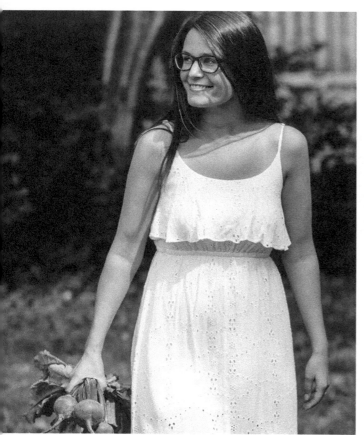
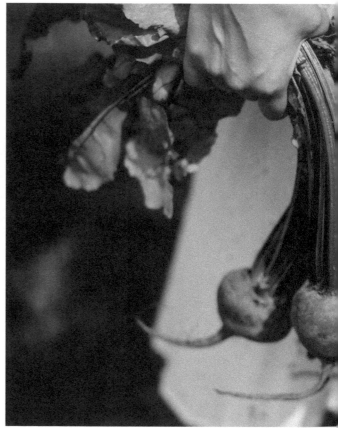

PHOTO CREDITS

All photos by Becki Peckham except photos on pages 42, 56, 59, 62, 67, 68, 73, 80, 83, 87, 99, 103, 108, 120, 123, and 124 by Jessica Mitton.

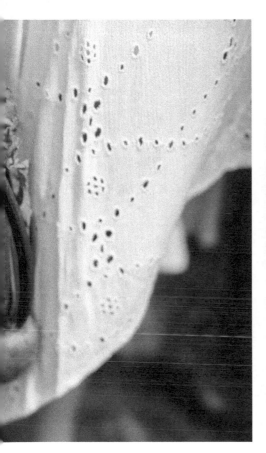
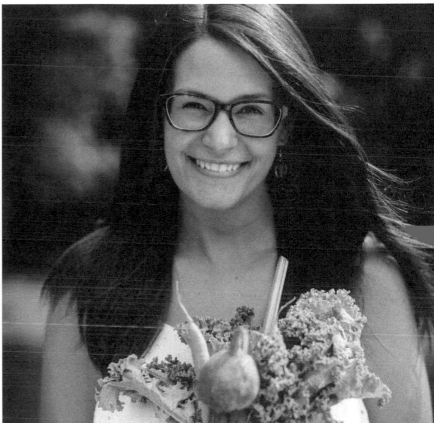

JESSICA MITTON is a Culinary Nutrition Expert and award-winning Certified Holistic Nutritional Consultant™ based in St. John's, Newfoundland. She has been featured in multiple publications and media channels, including the Academy of Culinary Nutrition's *From Scratch* cookbooks, CBC radio, and the national magazine *Optimyz*. When she is not busy creating in her kitchen, Jessica spends her time seeking out new adventures with her husband, Gareth.

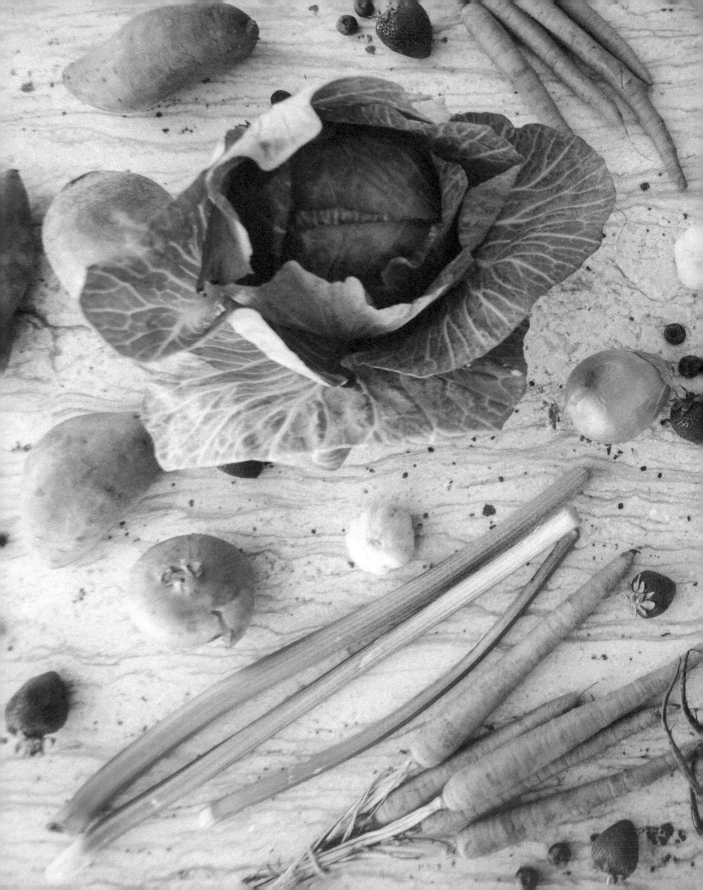

CPSIA information can be obtained
at www.ICGtesting.com
Printed in the USA
LVHW07s2034020818
585760LV00022B/420/P